Praise for *When Postpartum Packs a Punch*

"'First I had a baby. Then I felt crazy.' Such a powerful and poignant beginning to this important book on postpartum illness. What Kristina Cowan offers goes way beyond the courage of sharing her own and other personal stories. *When Postpartum Packs a Punch* speaks the language that postpartum families long for; it is rich with compassion, hope, and much-needed resources. This book is hugely informational, it is comforting, it is healing. "

Karen Kleiman, MSW, LCSW
Founder of The Postpartum Stress Center, and
author of Therapy and the Postpartum Woman
and The Art of Holding in Therapy

"If there was ever a book for fathers to educate themselves about perinatal mental health, it is this incredible book."

Mark Williams
Founder of International Fathers Mental Health Day,
speaker, author, and campaigner

"Are you feeling the punch of the postpartum period? Many new parents do. But in her book, *When Postpartum Packs a Punch*, Kristina Cowan helps the reader understand the scientific and personal sides of this often-unanticipated problem. This well-researched and well-written book can help you see that you are not alone in your struggle, and that there is help."

Dr. Jonathan S. Abramowitz
*Clinical psychologist, professor, and international
expert on OCD and anxiety disorders*

"Like a thunderclap on a cloudless day, perinatal mood and anxiety disorders upend a woman's vision of herself as a mother, as a person. With unflinching honesty, Kristina Cowan chronicles her odyssey through the heartbreak of depression following her son's birth. Using her story as a backdrop, Cowan weaves a tapestry of other women's voices, those who love them, and those who treat them. This enlightening book uniquely describes the history and development of international treatment models, which are finally being adopted and adapted in this country, serving up hope, inspiration, and reassurance."

Dr. Margaret Howard
*Director of the Day Hospital and Women's
Behavioral Health at Women and
Infants Hospital in Providence, Rhode Island*

"Kristina Cowan's book, *When Postpartum Packs a Punch: Fighting Back and Finding Joy,* is a great contribution to reliable education and research on perinatal mental health. As are most therapists and advocates, I am careful and protective when I recommend books to parents who are struggling with distress and trauma related to pregnancy, childbirth, and postpartum. I'm also determined to share evidence-based research in the field with providers and researchers. Cowan puts her expert reporting and expressive skills to work here, and the result is a resource that is informative, hopeful, and motivating. Including the subject of post-traumatic stress as a common perinatal mental health issue is just one example of the unique contributions in this book. We need more resources like this— using clear evidence to help families and providers improve the landscape for perinatal mental health. The information and personal excerpts empower families, as well as providers and policy makers. Together, and with solid information like this, we can make the landscape easier to travel, and our ability to care more effective. Cowan writes, 'Changing the way PMADs are discussed, both formally and informally, is crucial. ... By saying, "I've been where you are, and it's awful. But I got through it, and so will you," we show new mothers they're not alone. We offer hope, which is the heart of this book.'"

Wendy Newhouse Davis, Ph.D.
Counseling & Consultation, and executive director of Postpartum Support International

When POSTPARTUM Packs a Punch

Fighting Back and Finding Joy

Kristina Cowan

Praeclarus Press, LLC

www.PraeclarusPress.com

Praeclarus Press, LLC
2504 Sweetgum Lane
Amarillo, Texas 79124 USA
806-367-9950
www.PraeclarusPress.com

DISCLAIMER

The information contained in this publication is advisory only and is not intended to replace sound clinical judgment or individualized patient care. The author disclaims all warranties, whether expressed or implied, including any warranty as to the quality, accuracy, safety, or suitability of this informa-tion for any particular purpose.

ISBN: 978-1-946665-00-3

©2017 Kristina Cowan. All rights reserved.

Cover Design: Ken Tackett

Developmental Editing: Kathleen Kendall-Tackett

Copy Editing: Chris Tackett

Layout & Design: Nelly Murariu

A Note About Triggers: This book contains sensitive material and may trigger symp-toms of mood disorders. Please skip sections that might be upsetting to you until you believe you're ready for them, or consider having a friend or family member read for you.

A Note About Sources: Many of my sources throughout the book are people with whom I conducted interviews by phone, by Skype, in person, and electronically. I often had follow-up questions, so communication generally spanned a range of dates and forms. Timeframes for those interviews are mentioned in the first instance of the person's name, as a footnote. All other sources are listed as in-text citations, and may also be found in the References section at the back of the book.

For Noah and Syma,

the best parts of me

"I will not leave you comfortless: I will come to you."

JOHN 14:18
(KING JAMES VERSION)

Contents

Acknowledgments

The idea for this book was hatched as a prayer and a promise, in the earliest days of my encounter with postpartum depression. In those depths, I came closer to God than ever. If He hadn't heard my prayer—and held me to my promise to use my writing to help others—this book wouldn't exist. I'll always be grateful that He called and equipped me to write. It is the way I sing, pray, think, and spread hope. This book is proof that He works hard on our behalf, doing what only He can do: burnishing life's bad into a gilded glimpse of His glory.

I've been blessed by a troop of human help too. My strongest supporter has been my husband and best friend, Matt. He's made this project possible in *every* way, regularly reminding me that I could, in fact, get it done. Were it not for the two lives that have most changed mine, Noah and Syma, I wouldn't have developed an interest in perinatal mental health. Two sides of a golden coin, my children ushered in the fastest, most remarkable era of my life: motherhood.

During my research and reporting, I interviewed more mothers and fathers than I could ultimately include. Their stories of defeat, triumph, and enlightenment will be with me always. They're part of a survivor network key to saving and improving lives of other parents. The band of experts I called on—often more than once—graciously imparted their knowledge and perspective, adding depth and authority to my work. I'm especially grateful to Wendy Davis and Diana Barnes.

As a journalist, my closest allies are good editors, research, and the local library. They came through for me again on this project. Once I had words on paper, I entrusted them to a faithful band of critique partners: Anthony Trendl, Lori Mulligan Davis, Rachel Atkison, Christy Brunke, and Robin Melvin. They were with me through countless revisions and versions, and their insight and candor have made my writing sing. My editor-at-large, Kristin MacIntosh, helped me sort out editorial conundrums, always speedy and thoughtful in her replies. At the Naperville Public Library, Martha Mota lent a hand in acquiring articles and books vital to my research. Her kindness and efficiency shine.

Although I didn't realize it, my late mom, Karen, sowed in me all of the seeds I'd need to become a mother myself—love, forgiveness, and faith. I didn't have her for long, but she left me with an enduring legacy. My dad, who has read most everything I've written—including the rough drafts of this book—taught me two practical lessons: seek first an education, and work hard. They've served me well.

During my bout of postpartum depression, several family members and friends were instrumental in my healing, including my late brother, Jim McLaughlin; my aunt, Linda Sekerak; my mother-in-law, Sue Cowan; my late father-in-law, Paul Cowan; and my friends, Keme and Jamail Carter, and Janet and James Wolford. They didn't flinch, even when I shared my intrusive thoughts. They prayed without ceasing, and it made all the difference.

Last, but hardly least, I'm grateful to the kind friends who have cared for my little ones, keeping them safe and happy so I could write. Julie and Dave Oda and their family have loved Noah and Syma as their own. Their encouragement and prayers have energized me. And thanks to the late Denise Gallina, who enjoyed tending to my children during some of the final months of her life. Her love for them, her enthusiasm and support for my writing—these were invaluable as I finished the last chapters. I'll long be grateful for that special time.

List of Acronyms

CBT: cognitive behavioral therapy

CPN: community psychiatric nurse (in the UK)

DSM: *Diagnostic and Statistical Manual of Mental Disorders*

DSM-5: the 5th edition of the *Diagnostic and Statistical Manual of Mental Disorders*

ECT: electroconvulsive therapy

EMDR: eye movement desensitization and reprocessing

EPDS: Edinburgh Postpartum Depression Scale

ER: emergency room

LCSW: licensed clinical social worker

MBU: mother-baby unit or mother-and-baby unit

NICU: neonatal intensive care unit

OB/GYN: obstetrician-gynecologist

OCD: obsessive-compulsive disorder

PMAD: perinatal mood and anxiety disorder

PPA: postpartum anxiety

PPD: postpartum depression

PPND: paternal postnatal depression

PPOCD: postpartum obsessive-compulsive disorder

PSI: Postpartum Support International

PTSD: post-traumatic stress disorder

Foreword

Research confirms again and again women's psychiatric vulnerabilities during the childbearing years. However, cultural ideals about pregnancy and birth continue to overlook the psychological enormity of the transition to motherhood. Societal myths fail to recognize the transformative power of a woman's birth experience and its capacity not only to alter a woman's view of herself in the world, but to inform her thinking about herself as a mother.

Along with the practical elements of preparing for labor and delivery—hospital or home birth, midwife or obstetrician, epidural or no medical interventions unless necessary—generally comes a woman's anticipated vision of the birth experience that is infused with possibility and hopefulness, not only about the birth experience itself, but about her very future with that unborn child. That vision is frequently crafted during pregnancy, and sometimes even years before conception. It is affected by women's circumstances, their relationships with their partners and family members, along with what they believe society expects of them in the role of motherhood. When any part of that vision is chipped away, whether because of unforeseen events during labor or the unpredicted onset of a mood disorder during pregnancy or in the postpartum period, what often remains is the searing pain of the inconceivable: the mismatch between expectations and reality.

It is this psychological contradiction that so often leaves women vulnerable to the downward spiral of depression and anxiety in the postpartum period. While the actual presentation of perinatal illness may look remarkably similar from woman to woman, embedded in women's symptoms are the individual and unique stories that so often go untold. Although conventional wisdom endorses the flawed idea that we recover from struggle and trauma by burying the story and our feelings, the only way we can truly make sense of our lived experiences is through the mechanism of story. It is the way we learn, and it is the way we heal. Sharing our stories has medicinal properties, not only for the courageous individuals who tell their stories, but for those who are privileged to hear them.

This is a book about the power of stories. Using her own personal story of birth and postpartum trauma as the backdrop for furthering our understanding of the breadth of perinatal mood and anxiety disorders, Kristina Cowan invites us into the lives and experiences of women who have so graciously shared their stories so that we, the readers, may find more meaning in our own. Simply identifying symptoms without understanding the historical context within which they occur can be isolating and stigmatizing. However, the sharing of stories connects us in the most profound of ways. While the details of these stories may be different, they are woven with the same emotional threads of anticipation and disappointment, frustration and disillusionment, expectation and sadness, anger and worry, pain and despair, hope and healing.

Throughout the following pages, Kristina skillfully links symptoms and risk factors to stories as she gives voice to women *and* men's authentic experiences of pregnancy and the postpartum period. In telling her personal birth story, she opens the door to a conversation about birth trauma and its close connection to the onset of perinatal illness. This is often overlooked because of our cultural insistence to create a halo around childbirth for all women, regardless of their birth experience. She addresses the many roads to wellness, outlining various treatment options and approaches. In addition, she lists many valuable resources where women and their families can turn for treatment and care.

Postpartum Support International's (PSI) organizational roots are founded in the extraordinary insight that emotional connection and social support are a requirement for healing from a pregnancy- or postpartum-related mood disorder. For years, PSI has been sharing a universal message with women and their families: "You are not to blame, you are not alone, and with proper treatment, you will get well." Telling stories of pain and healing empowers us, frees us, and joins us. As Kristina writes, "Postpartum depression was not part of my birth plan," but she says it has been life-changing. Having shared her story and the stories of others, she has become keenly aware that "it's only in sharing our stories, one by one, that we'll find lasting comfort and true healing."

Diana Lynn Barnes, Psy.D.

The Center for Postpartum Health

Editor, *Women's Reproductive Mental Health Across the Lifespan*

CHAPTER I

Nobody Told Me It Wouldn't Be Perfect

My Story of Postpartum Trauma

We need to be angels for each other, to give each other strength and consolation. Because only when we fully realize that the cup of life is not only a cup of sorrow but also a cup of joy will we be able to drink it.

HENRI J. M. NOUWEN,
Can You Drink the Cup?

First I had a baby. Then I felt crazy.

My first taste of motherhood was hardly the honeyed bliss women dream about. My son, Noah, arrived in March 2009 on the heels of a complicated birth that left me injured. A day after I brought my baby home, I was in the emergency room. Wracked by pain worse than childbirth, I believed I might die and strand my child.

A week later, I started crying. I couldn't stop. I couldn't always explain the tears, even to myself. My head swelled with images of the baby plummeting down the trash chute. I wanted my old life back, the one where I was in control.

The idea of being labeled an unfit mother troubled me. Someone would surely take Noah away from me. More troubling was what might happen if I did nothing. Would I get worse—hallucinate, maybe, or fall far from reality? My fear of the unknown trumped my fear of stigma, so I sought help. First, I prayed. My prayers were mostly nonverbal, tear-soaked pleas. I read from the Book of Psalms. I asked for prayer from those closest to me, and tabled my writing career. My mental and physical health had to come first. I needed to sleep. I wanted to exercise.

After a few weeks, I called my OB/GYN and shared my symptoms. Above all, I said I was scared. I didn't feel like myself. She quickly treated me for postpartum *something*. She prescribed antidepressants and referred me to a talk therapist. At first it wasn't obvious what I was fighting. Later, it was clear I had symptoms of a perinatal mood and anxiety disorder (PMAD). I doubted anything could make me well—not medicine, and not God.

I was wrong.

Soon, my body and mind were on the mend, and I shared my story with my husband, friends, and family. Talking is a form of therapy, even when it's informal, and as long as the listener is interested. So I kept talking. I wanted to get well for my child, my husband, and myself. The seeds of my healing were rooted in those conversations. Others said hearing about my trials put them at ease to share theirs—in some cases, for the first time. They were empowered by relating their stories, and I knew I wasn't alone.

Some nights, I would fall asleep imagining Jesus, a towering figure sitting in a rocking chair, and I would grab his hand. In the past, when others spoke of such tactics, I figured they were zealots or weak-minded. Now I realized that, like me, they had reached the end of themselves. Admitting I needed God's help was akin to walking out on a tightrope stretched over a canyon, and the only thing that steadied me was my faith. I was supposed to be a parent, but I felt like a child, desperately leaning and some-what blind. In that darkness, I collided with the generosity and compassion of God's spirit. Only suffering could have sent me to those glorious depths.

What's at the Heart of This Book?

The better I felt, the more clearly I understood what happened: the physical and mental trauma I faced during childbirth, and the days just after, triggered my mood disorder. I wondered if others had similar encounters. I revealed my story within my small social circle, and discovered that several women had either dealt with birth trauma, mood disorders, or both. I had known some of the women for years, but I didn't know what they endured after childbirth. If the women I knew hid their troubles, surely women in the general population had done the same. I suspected birth trauma and mood disorders were far more pervasive than most people considered them to be.

I wanted to find out.

I would ask more questions, conduct formal interviews, and do extensive research—all second nature to me as a journalist.

Why wasn't there a book offering the sort of encouragement I gathered from others? It certainly would help. Holding a book in my hands with testimonies from others would be proof that I wasn't dreaming up my illness, and that I was part of a larger community. Such a book could help others, too. So I set to writing it. The result rests within these pages: the book I wanted, but couldn't find, one that explores stories of birth trauma and mood disorders, and offers solace.

As I expanded my research to the general population—and after having my second child, with no trauma or mood disorder—I came to believe that childbirth is naturally violent, even if no physical or mental upset are involved.

There is no graceful, easy way to extract a mini-human being from its mother's womb. She must bear a series of internal explosions, also known as contractions, sometimes for hours on end. Not unlike a soldier in combat, she's vulnerable and faces uncertainties. The stakes are life-and-death. She's saddled with gear, in the form of monitors and needles, and possibly pumped full of medication that may or may not agree with her system. Even without interventions, such as forceps or an emergency cesarean section, she braves a unique battlefield.

Though my story is woven throughout this book, its core lies in the words of the mothers and fathers I have interviewed. They're diverse in their backgrounds and perspectives, and their voices underscore the prevalence of mood disorders after childbirth. They show how an overcoming spirit can fight terrors of the mind, and win.

The book is divided into three parts. Part One covers the different PMADs, Part Two focuses on healing and recovery, and Part Three looks at the progress we've made in treating PMADs, and the work we have yet to accomplish. In addition to stories from parents, experts weigh in with their perspectives and experiences, and research is included throughout.

Each parent I spoke with navigated a different path to well-ness. Some women called on their husbands, friends, and family. Others relied on therapists, medicine, or alternative remedies. Still, others pointed to mothers' groups, churches, or their faith as key. While each situation was unique, the women and men agreed that increased awareness is necessary to fight the illnesses and their stigma.

Two areas of the book are of particular importance to me: Chapter 6, on stigma, and Chapter 7, on husbands/partners. Western culture gives little more than a superficial nod—if that— to these subjects. Perinatal mood disorders are treatable illnesses, yet most cases are overlooked and untreated. Why? Stigma is one of the culprits. Women don't seek help out of fear they'll be labeled "crazy" or "bad mothers." Because spouses/partners are a new mother's first line of defense, they should know the warning signs for mood disorders, and what to do if they suspect she's struggling. Men also need to set up support for themselves and ask for help, because they too can get PMADs.

It took me more than a year to reach a place I considered solid emotional ground. Not all mothers are as fortunate. Some suffer silently. In the rare-but-worst cases, they take their own lives and/or their children's. One way to stem this plague is in sharing stories—our own, and those of women we love. By saying, "I've been where you are, and it's awful. But I got through it, and so will you," we show new mothers they're not alone. We offer hope, which is the heart of this book.

My Story

My pregnancy with Noah was uncomplicated. We were healthy, as happy as two people sharing one body can be. I opted to induce labor 3 days before he was due. I wanted my OB, who was on call that day, to deliver him.

Picking a date to have my baby offered me the illusion of being in control. It put me at ease until the night before, when I couldn't sleep. I greeted induction day in a haze of nervous exhaustion. Soon after my husband, Matt, and I arrived at the Chicago hospital at 7 a.m., we learned I was already in the early stages of labor. To speed things along, the nurse hooked me up to a stream of Pitocin, a synthetic hormone that spurs labor (Weiss, 2016).

For the first few hours, the contractions were mild. Then, in what seemed to be an instant, they swelled to severe. Squatting and rocking to ease the pain, a slow panic crept over me. I had a *human being* inside of me. My body would have to contort and squeeze him out. But I felt as stiff as the icebergs lining Lake Michigan outside my hospital window.

I needed a strong dose of help.

I summoned the nurse and requested an epidural. It was a good move. Soon, I was ready to push. Three hours later, I was still pushing, with little sensation or progress. I hadn't eaten in 12 hours. The hormone-and-medicine cocktail that swirled in my body made me vomit. I was on the brink of fainting, and the baby's heart rate fell some. My doctor suggested forceps. She assured Matt and me that a simple nudge would loosen the baby. An emergency C-section would be a last resort.

I trusted my doctor and agreed to the forceps.

A new, unfamiliar team descended on my room, including extra nurses and an anesthesiologist who boosted my epidural. The spike in drugs made me feel as if I were floating. I was strangely calm as I watched the doctor and a medical student lower two mammoth metal prongs into my body. They clamped and jostled my son's head, gashing his cheek and one of his ears. I pushed. The doctors pulled. Noah was born. Full of relief when I saw that he was okay, I exhaled. My physical torture was over—or so I thought. With the labor medication still in my system, I started postpartum painkillers. The sheer excitement of it all, amplified by the drugs, sent me into a satisfied daze.

I had sustained a 3rd-degree tear from the forceps, but the doctors and nurses didn't explain what it might mean for me physically. In a dreamy state of ignorance, I sailed from delivery to recovery, celebrating Noah's healthy, dramatic arrival. Family called. Friends visited. Our joy multiplied. We had created a mini-us, one who existed only because of our union. We reveled in new-parent euphoria.

Not for long.

Though I was supposed to be in the hospital for 48 hours following the birth, I was ushered out after 36, because another mother needed the room. Besides, a nurse said, I'd be happier at home. Soon after returning to our high-rise apartment, my body failed. My bladder and bowels shut down, and I ballooned with fluid. Several times I called my OB, who suggested laxatives. They didn't work. In the wee hours, Matt and I headed to the ER. We brought our 3-day-old Noah, because no family had yet arrived to help look after him.

Inside the busy ER, a staffer started my paperwork. Eyeing Noah in his stroller, she said, "I wouldn't have my infant in here if I were you. All these germs? He could get sick."

I already was afraid that my condition would worsen, and I would die. Now I imagined Noah dying too. Tears streamed down my cheeks. She apologized and hustled to get us into a private waiting room.

Another ER attendant noticed that I was crying, and assumed we were there for Noah.

"What's wrong with your baby?" she asked.

"Nothing. He's perfect," I said. "I'm a mess, and I haven't learned how to pump milk yet. I'm worried that once the doctors see me here, my body won't be available to nurse him. What if he wakes up? He'll starve."

She ordered a breast pump and helped me learn to pump milk. I filled four ounces into a bottle, which is enough for a feeding. I clung to this small victory. Although Noah was asleep, he hadn't eaten in a few hours. If he did wake up, at least he would have food.

Even so, I worried. While I was pregnant, friends and family mentioned that if infants took a bottle or pacifier too soon, they might not readily return to the breast (a condition known as "nipple confusion"; Moreland & Coombs, 2000). I wanted to nurse him as long as possible, and avoid bottles and formula. Reflecting on this now, I'm comforted. Despite the fright of my first days as a parent, I didn't lose hold of the finer points of Noah's well-being. My mothering instincts were intact.

As 2 more hours passed, we waited. Induced labor was easy, by comparison. I limped to and from the bathroom, seeking but not finding relief. My abdomen and lower back felt like a war zone, with fiery darts streaking from side to side.

Once the doctor arrived, she asked a nurse to drain my bladder. To the great surprise of us all, it held more than twice the amount considered full. It would be trickier to relax my bowels. The doctor tried to loosen them manually—the worst, most humiliating pain of my life—and sent me home with orders to take more laxatives.

Later that morning, Matt drove me three blocks to my OB's office, and I struggled to sit upright, preferring instead the fetal position. Jolted by my ashen appearance, my doctor said, "This isn't your fault. We need to blame someone, so let's blame me."

She explained that the trauma caused by the 3rd-degree tear made it difficult for me to go to the bathroom. The injury ultimately caused my bladder and bowels to stop working. She hooked me up to a transportable catheter, and instructed me to buy a few enemas, go home, and sit in a warm bath.

Her formula worked.

Three days later, my body was functioning and on the mend. But my emotions started to crumble. I feared something would happen to Noah. What if he fell down the trash chute? What if I hit him on the head with a frying pan? I thought my husband would discover that I was a terrible wife and mother, grow to hate me, and leave.

I rode a hormonal seesaw, crying at moments that would otherwise elicit a smile, such as when my father-in-law called to check on us, when a little girl on the street waved at me, when one of my clients sent a baby gift.

Worst of all, I saw myself as a failure. By inducing early, I had rushed my child into the world before he was ready. I wasn't able to give birth the "right" way. Now my mind was a coil of dark thoughts.

Silent suffering isn't my style. I didn't hide my tears. I shared my intrusive thoughts, as they're called, with my husband, and with our families and friends. Eventually I called my OB. She was warm, nonjudgmental, and swift to act. Within a few days, I was taking antidepressants and visiting a therapist. The therapy went a long way to restoring my jilted sense of self-worth. The medicine quelled the constant crying. It also cast me onto an emotional tundra, and froze my capacity for laughter, tears, or any strong emotion.

I stopped taking the antidepressants after 4 months, and wrapped up therapy at the same time. A few months later, I thought my postpartum depression had reappeared. I developed a rash of unusual symptoms—fatigue, aching joints, and unexplained irritability. Some days, my attention crept down the dark alleys of memory. I would cry as I thought of how my parents had been mean-spirited to one another during their divorce. As their child, I wondered if I had a cruelty gene. Would I too hurt my own child and husband?

I went back to my OB, the doctor I trusted most. She ordered blood work to test my thyroid, and results showed it was imbalanced. I sought the help of an endocrinologist, who determined that as a result of the pregnancy, I had developed Hashimoto's disease, an autoimmune disorder. With Hashimoto's, the immune system attacks the thyroid gland, disrupting its ability to produce hormones. Over time, this leads to an underactive thyroid, also known as hypothyroidism, which slows down all of the body's processes, including brain function, heart rate, and metabolism. It can even mimic depression (Office on Women's Health, 2012).

I started medication to restore my thyroid shortly before Noah turned 1. Six months later, I felt much better. Treatment and time stitched my frayed ends, but I was fundamentally changed. Parts of me are stronger. Parts of me are still broken and messy. That's long been true. But motherhood forced me to admit it.

I'm glad.

It was easier to carry the weight of Noah's little life once I fessed up to my many imperfections.

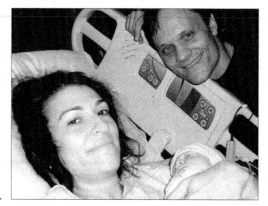

Now we are three: Matt, Noah, and me on the night Noah was born, March 2, 2009, in Chicago.

Unqualified

Perinatal mood disorders are like yeast devouring sugar. They feast on an emotional hardship in a woman's life and ominously rise, dominating her daily existence. In my case, the emotional sugars were related to my tendency to be an overachiever, and the early loss of my mother. Yet, the feeding frenzy was ultimately a good thing. It forced me to confront issues I would've just as soon swept into a dark corner.

The unraveling of my self-worth started with the forceps delivery, the trip to the ER, and uncontrollable crying spells. A capable mother would have done better. I thought of myself as Hester Prynne in *The Scarlet Letter* (Hawthorne, 2011), with a red emblem stamped on my chest, only mine was an "F," for failure, instead of Hester's "A," for adultery. If the people around me knew how inept I was, they would snatch Noah and send me away.

Self-flagellation powered my mood disorder and hurled me into a shadowy netherworld reigned by dark thoughts. I hunted for reasons why I was worthy of reproach. Digging into my past, I found them. My parents divorced when I was 8 years old, and my mother died when I was 15. Memories of a nuclear family and a loving mother were dim. How could I furnish Noah with these things so vital to a happy childhood?

I felt unqualified to be a mother.

Until Noah, I had spent life *qualifying*: for college, graduate school, reporting and editing jobs, and my freelance career. Overachieving was my lifestyle. Hope Edelman, who has written extensively about women who lose their mothers early in life, says,

> These behaviors develop and persist because we can convince ourselves that they aid us in some way. ... A girl becomes an overachiever to elicit the praise and respect from strangers that she can't get

from her family, or to force her surviving parent to acknowledge her success (1994, pp. 170-171).

I even tried to be an overachiever while I was pregnant with Noah, and assumed if I did everything right, I would succeed in motherhood. I followed my doctor's suggestions, read baby books, and took parenting classes. I avoided things that could harm the baby, and exercised constantly, right up to the eve of his birth.

The mushier side of motherhood—things like preparing a nursery, cooing at tiny clothes and shoes, soaking up the limelight at baby showers—annoyed me. I preferred to focus on my journalism career, so I took as many writing assignments as possible. Sitting with a group of friends a few days before Noah's arrival, I revealed my biggest concerns: fitting the baby into my busy work schedule and finding a nanny. I relegated parenting to a post on the outskirts of my life.

Pushing to excel at the mechanics of pregnancy, staying buried in work—I used these to distance myself from painful emotions I associated with losing my mother, and fears I had about becoming a mother. Noah's birth erased the distance. In his book, *Glorious Ruin: How Suffering Sets You Free,* Tullian Tchividjian says, "Nothing forces us to confront the deeper questions of life quite like suffering. Nothing makes us face the gnawing emptiness inside more nakedly. Nothing confirms our suspicion more powerfully that this is *not* how things are supposed to be" (2012, p. 17).

Buckling under the weight of mental and emotional tumult— this isn't how new motherhood is supposed to be. My mood disorder was a mantle I didn't want. Surely it meant I was a bad person. Consoling me on the phone one day soon after Noah was born, my brother, Jim, said, "This is not *who* you are. It's *where* you are." I knew he was right. I had to push through the pain. But it would be a while before I believed my plight wasn't a personal failing.

A Mother Lost, A Mother Born

Did I really have to mourn my mother all over again, 20 years after she died? At first, I didn't see what good could come from it.

When my mother died, I was a teenager, lacking an adequate emotional reserve to help me make sense of her death. I forged ahead because I had to, and learned to live—happily, even—without her. In some ways, the loss made me stronger and more determined to chase my goals. In other ways, I felt unworthy, questioning if God had allowed her passing to punish me for being a bratty child. Was I less deserving than my friends who had their mothers? I contemplated this, particularly at major milestones like graduating from college and getting married.

Motherhood was different. It was worse.

More than ever, I needed the unconditional love and acceptance only my mother could give me. I needed her in the delivery room, in the ER, during the crying spells, and when I was trying to determine if I should take antidepressants. She should have been with me.

I was also suddenly aware that someone else would be influenced by her absence, even if he didn't know it: my child. Not only was he without a maternal grandma, he would be sorely affected by the shortcomings I had as a motherless woman. My model for mothering long gone, I worried that I wouldn't know how to be a good mother, or how to offer him the emotional support he would need. He too would suffer.

My reaction to the loss of my mother was a STUG, a Subsequent, Temporary Upsurge of Grief (Edelman, 2007). I had walked through life *knowing* if I had children, they would miss out on knowing her. It was quite different to become a mother and suddenly *feel* my loss compounded by my child's loss. The STUG helped me grieve for my mother in my new role as a mother, something I would have to do sooner or later.

In adulthood, major events like becoming a mother can take a woman to a new level of awareness for what she's lost in her mother, Edelman says:

Instead of being labeled pathological, as they once were, STUGs are now considered universal for bereaved persons, especially those who lost a parent at an early age. They're also considered beneficial in the long term. Because STUGs allow women to work on the loss from new and different angles over time, they're considered a healthy mechanism for working through grief (2007, p. 5).

Long talks with my therapist, friends, family, and especially my husband, allowed me to deal with thoughts and feelings. I began to accept that part of me would forever be sad about my children not knowing my mother. Still, my sadness can coexist with the joy motherhood brings, and even complement it. Grief is a lifelong process. I won't "get over" losing my mother, but I can live to honor her and continue her legacy.

I've been surprised to find parenthood reconnecting me with my mother. I often talk and act the way she did with me when I was a child, remembering her traditions and beliefs. Her influence, though brief, is embedded in the deepest part of me. Motherhood has helped me reclaim part of my mother, for my family and myself.

The Value of Pain

For better or worse, pain is powerful. Madeleine L'Engle, in her book, *Walking on Water: Reflections on Faith and Art*, says, "Pain is not always creative; received wrongly, it can lead to alcoholism and madness and suicide. Nevertheless, without it we do not grow" (2001, p. 68).

Initially, my postpartum pain felt more like a steamroller than an agent of growth. I mentioned earlier how my first days of motherhood were the first time I felt unqualified for something.

This was a painful admission, especially for a perfectionist. But on that emotional ground zero, I could build from scratch. I grew to believe that I couldn't fix everything on my own, and that I could ask for help. I grew to understand that God didn't grant me a beautiful baby and the gift of motherhood because He thought I would perform flawlessly. If anything, He tapped me because I was an unlikely candidate. These were healthy realizations. L'Engle writes,

> In a very real sense not one of us is qualified, but it seems that God continually chooses the most unqualified to do his work, to bear his glory. If we are qualified, we tend to think that we have done the job ourselves. If we are forced to accept our evident lack of qualification, then there's no danger that we will confuse God's work with our own, or God's glory with our own (2001, p. 67).

The events surrounding Noah's birth and my postpartum depression forced me to acknowledge my lack of qualifications. When I reflect on that time, I credit the hand of God with getting me through it. I was covered by love, from the generous baby meals sent by friends and family, to the compassionate bedside manner of my OB, to the many willing to listen as I recounted my traumatic childbirth and trip to the ER. Time, medicine, and a therapist helped my mind heal. God had surrounded me with everything and everyone I needed to cope and recover.

The best part of new motherhood, chaos and all, was that it became a window through which I glimpsed God's glory.

My healing came full circle with the arrival of my second child, a girl named Syma, 2 ½ years after Noah. The pregnancy and birth were uncomplicated. She was born naturally, 3 days after her due date and without an induction. I refused Pitocin and squeezed her out after three short pushes. Knowing that women with a history of perinatal mood disorders are more prone to them with subsequent children, I braced for more anguish. When it didn't come, I was surprised and thankful.

I had stumbled upon the name Syma in my early 20s. One of my first bosses often mentioned her sister named Syma, which she said was Hebrew for "joy." I decided it would be the name I'd use if I ever had a daughter. A few months before she was born, I researched the name, and found it defined instead as "flourishing" or "treasure." No matter, I thought; to me, it still meant joy. Then I chose her middle name, Amaris, which means "God has promised." I picked "Syma Amaris," not just for its lilt, but because it symbolized my faith in God's promise of joy. Psalm 30 says, "Weeping may last through the night, but joy comes with the morning." Thanks to my children, I experienced the full weight of that verse.

Syma's arrival gave me a new perspective on Noah's birth: though steeped in trauma, it was beautiful. I couldn't see beauty in the individual moments as I lived through them. But time and a second birth enabled me to distill something sweet from an unsavory situation, to appreciate it in all of its uncommon splendor.

I'm grateful for my first days as a mother. They brought healing from wounds I didn't know I had. They nudged me toward a partnership with God, one where I'm getting to know Him better. Should I somehow forget I need God's help, my children are faithful reminders.

My story is but one illustration of a battle braved by many women and their families. Some have shared their journeys with me, revealing how mood disorders play out differently from person to person. Discovering the sheer volume of families affected by these illnesses, we should be startled into acknowledging this as a major health epidemic and stirred to action.

CHAPTER 2

A Different Kind of War

When Childbirth Leads to Post-Traumatic Stress

The conflict between the will to deny horrible events and the will to proclaim them aloud is the central dialectic of psychological trauma.

JUDITH HERMAN,
Trauma and Recovery

A doctor reading the clinical file on my first experience of childbirth would probably consider it routine. But for me, it was hardly standard. It left me feeling violated, misled, and with a great sense of loss.

Because I had signed up for an induction, my OB arranged for a midwife to break my water, to help keep labor on a steady course (for a detailed account of my story, see Chapter 1). Though I had wanted it to rupture on its own, I didn't speak up. I assumed my doctor knew best. The midwife was kind and just doing her job, but my baby, who'd been calm until then, shuddered and twisted. This unwanted procedure unnerved both of us. I perceived it as an invasion of my body, something that violated what I believed was best for my baby. Because I didn't voice my concerns, the scene haunted me.

Later, a nurse impassively offered that I might be in labor for a while. Most inductions lasted at least 24 hours, she added, and often led to C-sections. Her words danced around the room like bright-red bursts of exclamation. Why hadn't my OB mentioned this? Equipped with that information, I wouldn't have signed up for an induction. I felt misled by my doctor.

Perhaps the most devastating part of Noah's birth was my sense of loss. The intensity of the drugs used to support the forceps left me physically and emotionally numb—so it seemed as if I was watching the birth happen to someone else. I still mourn the loss of being fully alert and feeling the moment when my first child made his first trip, from my womb to the outside world.

In hindsight, trauma stormed the stage where Noah's birth played out. Eventually, that trauma also had a starring role in my story of postpartum depression.

What are Perinatal Mood and Anxiety Disorders?

Postpartum depression often is used as an umbrella term for the different anxiety and mood disorders associated with childbirth. Though it's just one of the disorders, many people have at least heard of it. Still, they might not understand the specifics, especially if they haven't experienced it, or know someone who has. Mainstream media tends to focus on extreme cases, such as Andrea Yates (Belluck, 2014), where a mother harms her child/children, or herself. TV news coverage, for instance, highlights the horror of it all, and eclipses important details worth knowing. For instance, Yates suffered from postpartum psychosis—not postpartum depression. Psychosis is relatively rare, and many who experience it don't harm their children or themselves: they get treatment, they recover, and they go on to lead productive lives.

Unless we make these distinctions between psychosis and postpartum depression, and educate others about *all* perinatal mood disorders, the public will continue to draw incorrect conclusions from well-publicized cases. It's as easy as it is unfair to transfer those assessments to other women. Walling them in with our own suspicions and fears, we treat them as if they're a threat to their children, themselves, or both. By doing so, we give stigma an undeserved license to continue silencing women. Afraid of being branded as crazy, unfit mothers, they don't speak up and get the help they need. They often get worse, and their families languish as a result.

It's a senseless spiral: sensationalized cases breed misinformation, which drives stigma that holds women captive, and bars them from getting medical attention. To break this pattern, we must first pull apart the sometimes-confusing terminology of perinatal mood and anxiety disorders (PMADs), and offer clear, simple definitions.

PMADs can surface during pregnancy, or up to a year after childbirth. During pregnancy they're called prenatal, antenatal, or antepartum. After a baby is born, they're dubbed postpartum or postnatal. Some mothers develop more than one, so it's important to be aware of the various symptoms and risk factors, and how common they are. Below is a list of five major PMADs:

▸ **Prenatal/postpartum depression (PPD)** can involve feelings of anger, sadness, irritability, guilt, lack of interest in the baby, changes in eating and sleeping habits, trouble concentrating, hopelessness, and sometimes, thoughts of harming the baby or oneself.

▸ **Prenatal/postpartum anxiety (PPA)** may be characterized by extreme worries and fears, often about the baby's health and safety. Some women have panic attacks, shortness of breath, chest pain, dizziness, a feeling of losing control, and numbness and tingling.

▸ **Prenatal/postpartum obsessive-compulsive disorder (OCD)** might include repetitive, upsetting, and unwanted thoughts or mental images, known as obsessions. A woman also may have compulsions, where she does certain things over and over to reduce the anxiety caused by the unwanted thoughts. She is extremely disturbed by the thoughts, and very unlikely to ever act on them.

▸ **Postpartum post-traumatic stress disorder (PTSD)** is often caused by a traumatic or frightening childbirth, or past trauma, particularly sexual abuse. Symptoms can include flashbacks to the trauma, with feelings of anxiety, and the need to avoid things related to the event.

▸ **Postpartum psychosis (PP)** is a break with reality. Women might see and hear voices or images that others can't, called hallucinations. They may believe things that aren't true and distrust those around them. They can encounter periods of confusion and memory loss, and seem manic. Though it's relatively rare, psychosis is a severe, dangerous condition that needs immediate attention (Postpartum Support International, n.d.).

I take a closer look at each of these in the chapters ahead, through real-life cases, research, and expert perspectives. From this point, I use "PMAD," "perinatal mood and anxiety disorder," and "perinatal mood disorder" as general terms to refer to the different illnesses.

Two other conditions I won't explore in-depth are postpartum stress syndrome (PSS) and bipolar mood disorder.

About one in five women experience PSS, the most common postpartum emotional reaction, but it isn't as severe as postpartum depression. It involves feelings of anxiety, self-doubt, and a strong desire to be a perfect mother. Some women with postpartum stress syndrome develop clinical depression, but others don't (Kleiman & Raskin, 2013).

Postpartum-depression expert Karen R. Kleiman[1] explains that PSS is synonymous with the term "adjustment disorder," as defined by the 5th edition of the *Diagnostic and Statistical Manual of Mental Disorders (DSM-5)*. The *DSM-5* says that adjustment disorders are characterized by "emotional or behavioral symptoms in response to an identifiable stressor." The stressor could be one event, or more than one (American Psychiatric Association, 2013).

"Women with PSS generally don't need medication, and may or may not need or want therapy," says Kleiman, founder of The Postpartum Stress Center in Pennsylvania, a treatment and

---

[1] My personal communication with Karen Kleiman took place between January 16, 2014, and July 21, 2014.

professional training center for prenatal and postpartum depression and anxiety. In treating PSS patients, she makes sure they're sleeping well, connecting with their partner, and maybe joining support groups for mothers. "We see a lot of women who don't have clinical depression, but would have an adjustment disorder."

Bipolar mood disorder involves two phases: lows and highs. The lows are called depression, and the highs are known as mania or hypomania. Many women are diagnosed for the first time with bipolar depression or mania while they're pregnant, or postpartum. The disorder may appear as a severe depression, so women need evaluation and follow-up on past and current mood changes and cycles to determine if there's a bipolar dynamic (Postpartum Support International, n.d.).

The rest of this chapter examines trauma and postpartum PTSD. I focus first on this topic because threads of trauma run through all mood disorders. A traumatic birth, for instance, might lead to a mood disorder, and the illness itself is a form of trauma. An increased knowledge of trauma enables us to acknowledge how common it is. Recognizing the commonality will, ideally, help us release our fears of admitting that at some point—even with the births of our beloved children—we endure trauma.

Dr. Bessel A. van der Kolk, an international expert on post-traumatic stress since the 1970s, offers a clear explanation of what it means to be traumatized:

> In the long term, the largest problem of being traumatized is that it's hard to feel that anything that's going on around you really matters. It is difficult to love and take care of people and get involved in pleasure and engagements because your brain has been re-organized to deal with danger. It is only partly an issue of consciousness. Much has to do with unconscious parts of the brain that keep

interpreting the world as being dangerous and frightening and feeling helpless. You know you shouldn't feel that way, but you do, and that makes you feel defective and ashamed (Bullard, 2014).

Birth Trauma: "In the Eye of the Beholder"

To my doctors and nurses, my son's birth appeared routine. For me, it was far from what I had imagined. My plans and expectations were dashed. The complications—especially the trip to the ER—were the worst things I had experienced. They spelled trauma and sowed the seeds of postpartum depression.

Dr. Cheryl Tatano Beck,[2] an expert on postpartum post-traumatic stress disorder (PTSD), and Board of Trustees Distinguished Professor at the University of Connecticut's School of Nursing, conducted research that points to such a disconnect between women and their care providers. "What a mother perceives as birth trauma may be seen quite differently through the eyes of obstetric care providers, who may view it as a routine delivery and just another day at the hospital," according to Beck's 2004 study (p. 28). The study examined what women view as traumatic during childbirth that could lead to postpartum PTSD.

Reflecting on Noah's birth and the care I received, I believe my body and my trust were violated:

▸ I didn't receive all of the pertinent information about how difficult inductions can be.

▸ Although I agreed to the forceps, I wasn't expecting them. They were foreign objects inserted into my body

---

2   My personal communication with Dr. Cheryl Tatano Beck took place between September 1, 2015, and September 21, 2015.

with force. In a sense, they too had violated me by injuring me and leaving gashes on my newborn's face.

▶ No one explained what a 3rd degree tear meant, or warned me there could be complications.

▶ The hospital discharged us early, and failed to determine how well my body was functioning.

Someone else might not have been fazed, but I was. Why? Because, as Beck's study shows, "birth trauma is in the eye of the beholder" (2004, p. 32). According to the study,

> The concept of birth trauma involves traumatic experiences that may occur during any phase of childbearing. During any phase, the trauma may be classified as a negative outcome including a stillbirth, an obstetric complication (e.g., an emergency cesarean), or psychological distress (fear of an epidural) (Beck, 2004, p. 32).

List of Birth Traumas

Source: *Birth Trauma: In the Eye of the Beholder*, p. 32, by Dr. Cheryl Tatano Beck

▶ Stillbirth/infant death

▶ Emergency cesarean delivery/fetal distress

▶ Cardiac arrest

▶ Inadequate medical care

▶ Fear of epidural

▶ Congenital anomalies

▶ Inadequate pain relief

- ▸ Postpartum hemorrhage/manual removal of placenta
- ▸ Forceps/vacuum extraction/skull fracture
- ▸ Severe toxemia
- ▸ Premature birth
- ▸ Separation from infant in NICU
- ▸ Prolonged, painful labor
- ▸ Rapid delivery
- ▸ Degrading experience

Beck says women who perceive their births as traumatic are "systematically stripped of layers of protection—meaning women did not feel cared for, it was a dehumanizing process, they were stripped of their dignity, a lack of communication." She offers one image often related by those who have felt traumatized during childbirth: "[T]hey felt raped on the table, with everyone watching and no one helping."

Women in the study also reported that their expectations for labor-and-delivery care were shattered. Mothers described the care they received during delivery as mechanical, arrogant, cold, technical, and lacking empathy.

Dr. Michael W. O'Hara,[3] an expert on postpartum depression and psychology professor at the University of Iowa, says, "Almost anything that is perceived to be traumatic can create problems for a woman in the postpartum period." An important part of this is a violation of expectations. For example, he says, a forceps delivery isn't traumatic in principle, but a woman can perceive it to be so. He cited another, specific case: during a C-section, a woman's anesthesia didn't work, leading to severe pain, and she later developed PTSD.

---

3   My personal communication with Dr. Michael W. O'Hara took place between November 15, 2012, and October 22, 2015.

Perception is key, says Dr. Diana Lynn Barnes,[4] a psychotherapist who specializes in women's reproductive mental health: "If I think it's traumatic, it doesn't matter if my health care provider doesn't think so. Many women are very quick to doubt the reality of their own experience." According to a 2014 meta-analysis of 78 studies of postpartum PTSD:

Studies have shown that women's subjective experiences during labor and delivery are strongly associated with the development of PTSD due to childbirth (Czarnocka & Slade, 2000; Olde et al., 2005; Verreault et al., 2012). It is important to note that this may be and often is different from a medical provider's assessment of the childbirth experience. Further, a woman may go through a delivery that a physician may label as "normal" while the woman may assess her experience as traumatic (Grekin & O'Hara, p. 391).

Dr. Wendy N. Davis,[5] executive director of Postpartum Support International (PSI), a U.S.-based group that promotes awareness, prevention, and treatment of mental-health issues related to childbearing, has seen this tension play out. Davis, who leads trainings on perinatal mental health for care providers, once heard from a midwife confused by a mother referring to her birth as traumatic. The midwife had been present at the birth and didn't consider it traumatic, so Davis pointed her to Beck's eye-of-the-beholder study.

During a trauma, Davis says, people tend to shut down, so a mother may appear quiet and calm on the outside. If a woman is unable to fully express her questions and concerns as the trauma unfolds, PTSD can result. For a variety of reasons—confusion, uncertainty, fear—I didn't utter my questions during my son's

---

4 My personal communication with Dr. Diana Lynn Barnes took place between October 18, 2012, and June 19, 2016.

5 My personal communication with Dr. Wendy N. Davis took place between September 21, 2015, and February 23, 2016.

birth. This runs counter to how I usually operate. Looking back, I believe the birth trauma was so startling, I didn't know *how* to be my own best advocate. While I didn't contend with PTSD, the birth trauma I encountered was a trigger for postpartum depression.

Understanding Postpartum PTSD

Risk Factors, Prevalence, and Symptoms

Two groups of women are thought to be at increased risk for postpartum PTSD—those who experience trauma during childbirth, and those with past trauma not related to the birth (Grekin & O'Hara, 2014). Mothers who refer to childbirth as traumatic often will have faced unplanned interventions during labor and delivery, such as:

- an emergency C-section;

- a forceps- or vacuum-assisted vaginal delivery;

- the baby being sent to the neonatal intensive care unit (NICU);

- a severe physical complication, extreme pain, or injury related to pregnancy or childbirth, such as postpartum hemorrhage, unexpected hysterectomy, pre-eclampsia or eclampsia, a 3rd- or 4th-degree tear (for more on tears, see Chapter 1), or cardiac disease;

- feeling powerless, a lack of support and reassurance during the delivery, or that they weren't fully informed about what happens during childbirth; and/or

- a prolapsed umbilical cord (Grekin & O'Hara, 2014; Postpartum Support International, n.d.).

Those with past trauma may have been raped, sexually abused as children, or physically assaulted. "Among these women it is likely that PTSD symptoms were present before childbirth and simply continued into the postpartum period. It is also possible that the symptoms had resolved but were retriggered following childbirth" (Grekin & O'Hara, 2014, p. 390).

Dr. Sharon Dekel,[6] an assistant professor of psychology at Harvard Medical School, agrees that a history of trauma and PTSD put some at higher risk for developing PTSD after childbirth. She also points to a woman's "subjective appraisal" of childbirth as significant. But a combination of factors ultimately feed into the disorder. "It's not just an appraisal of the situation. It's who you are, your life experience, your support system, and other stressors in your life. It's difficult to predict who will have PTSD and who won't," Dekel explains.

Still, Grekin and O'Hara (2014) noted that researchers haven't consistently distinguished between the two different paths—birth-related or previous trauma—leading to the disorder. Research also has failed to differentiate between the types of study samples. Some researchers use samples from the community, while others use specific samples of individuals considered at-risk of developing the disorder. To present a more accurate picture, Grekin and O'Hara, in their 2014 meta-analysis do distinguish between the sample types, as well as what causes PTSD. Among the community samples, prevalence was 3 percent; at-risk populations had a much higher prevalence of 16 percent. In both the targeted and community samples, symptoms of postpartum depression "demonstrated the strongest association with postpartum PTSD" (2014, p. 397).

Beck has found this to be true in her research, as well: "One of the variables most correlated with elevated postpartum PTSD is

---

6   My personal communication with Dr. Sharon Dekel took place between November 6, 2015, and November 11, 2015.

postpartum depression." A woman screened for PPD should also be screened for PTSD, Beck says, but not many clinicians look for both. "Clinicians aren't as used to PTSD due to birth, so they screen for postpartum depression much more frequently than for PTSD." Beck was one of the authors of a 2011 report on PTSD in new mothers that suggests, "[W]hen women screen positive for postpartum depression, clinicians need to explore with new mothers if they are also experiencing any posttraumatic stress symptoms and vice-versa" (Beck et al., p. 226).

Dekel agrees. Because childbirth can lead to PTSD, it would be helpful to screen and educate women—especially those with a history of anxiety or symptoms of PTSD. "We [perform] a great service if we do more studies, if we try to understand who these women are."

It's important to know that birth trauma can lead to postpartum PTSD for some women, but not for others. Davis, of Postpartum Support International, says many with postpartum depression or postpartum anxiety are dealing with trauma, but they wouldn't receive a clinical diagnosis of postpartum PTSD. "I will often use the phrase, 'post-traumatic stress,' because I haven't diagnosed them with PTSD," Davis says. "There's a difference between PTSD and other trauma that doesn't result in PTSD. If we overuse PTSD, it loses its meaning."

Symptoms of the disorder may include:

▸ intrusive re-experiences of the past trauma, which might be the childbirth itself;

▸ flashbacks or nightmares;

▸ avoidance of things related to the event, including thoughts, feelings, people, places, and details;

▸ irritability, trouble sleeping, hypervigilance, exaggerated startle response;

- anxiety and panic attacks; and/or
- feeling detached and a sense of unreality (Postpartum Support International, n.d.).

Miles to Go

Postpartum PTSD is gaining increased attention among the medical and research communities. Dekel says it is "a new area of empirical investigation, in which data is derived from qualitative study of representative samples who are followed over time." The last 5 years have seen more studies on the topic, with groups from Europe and Australia leading the way. Dekel herself has studied PTSD in the general population, and she's now expanding her research, and conducting a study on the risk factors and incidence of the disorder after childbirth.

Significant work remains to better understand the disorder, and how to best serve the women who have it, according to Grekin and O'Hara (2014). For instance, risk factors that aren't straightforward should be investigated:

These factors include the individual experience of childbirth and the specific interactions that women have with medical staff during labor and delivery. It is necessary to understand what women view as negative experiences and interactions during childbirth, besides more objective factors such as medical complications or certain procedures (Grekin & O'Hara, 2014, p. 399).

Another area for future research is examining the long-term outcomes of the disorder's effects, and how they might pass from mother to child.

CHAPTER 2 - A DIFFERENT KIND OF WAR

Chrissy's Story

Some women, like Christina "Chrissy" McAlister,[7] endure trauma before childbirth and develop postpartum PTSD once they deliver a child. Before motherhood, Chrissy's life was rife with trauma. Her parents divorced when she was 4 years old, and her mother abandoned the family. Her father and paternal grandfather raised her from that point. At 9 years old, she joined Big Brothers Big Sisters of America, and was matched with a big sister. During her pre-teen years, she was inappropriately touched over the course of 2 years. In her teens, she sank into depression, spurred by the loss of a relationship with her mother. Medication, counseling, and her big sister helped her through it. Later, her best friend died in a car accident, and Chrissy was raped twice in college. "I have never had time to heal on everything that has happened in life. When I start to heal, something bad happens," she explains. Repeated devastation has cast her into perpetual fear of what lies ahead.

Chrissy's son was born in August 2013. For the first few weeks, she was happy and content. Around four weeks postpartum, "It became difficult for me to understand or even communicate my feelings well." The baby had jaundice and wasn't latching well during nursing, so she fought "to keep weight on him"—and found herself distraught over his health. Before the baby was born, Chrissy and her husband discussed how much she wanted to nurse. Knowing this, he pressured her to continue, so she pumped milk every 2 ½ hours. The rigorous pumping and stress of it all led to sleepless nights. Her milk supply dwindled, and she lost her appetite. She explains, "We had to bottle-feed him formula supplementation, because I wasn't producing enough milk. That's when I became angry, and felt I was missing out on the bonding time with my son." She was left feeling detached from the baby. "I felt like a failure. Then I got really sick."

---

7 My personal communication with Christina McAlister took place between July 16, 2015, and January 4, 2016.

When her son was a little over a month old, she tried to pump and fell into an unstoppable shaking spell. It was the middle of the night, so her husband took her to the emergency room. She assumed she would improve in another week or two, and didn't give the ER care providers the details of her feelings: "They wanted me to talk, but I didn't know what to talk about. I didn't refuse. I just said, 'I don't know what's wrong.'"

But her symptoms worsened when she went home. "I just paced around my house. I stopped eating. I didn't sleep. I didn't feel beautiful anymore," she says. "I found myself consumed with fear, embarrassment, and shame. Not because of anything I had done. I felt these emotions because of society's stigma towards mental illness, especially postpartum depression."

Eventually, Chrissy's husband insisted she get help, and they scheduled an emergency appointment with her OB/GYN. She agreed to be voluntarily hospitalized. This landed her in an ambulance, strapped down as she headed to the mental-health ward of a hospital 30 minutes from her home. Doctors and nurses monitored her behavior closely. After 2 days of pacing the hallways, attending group meetings, and not eating, she was diagnosed with bipolar disorder, and started seeing a psychiatrist and a counselor, but neither of them specialized in maternal mental health. She was prescribed anti-anxiety medication and sleeping pills, which helped her sleep. "I knew I wasn't bipolar and that something else was wrong with me. The doctors and my husband were not listening to me. Was I really losing my mind just because I had a baby that I had prepared for and wanted so badly?" The only upside of being hospitalized was the highly structured environment. She attended groups throughout the day that taught her coping skills, and met others with mental struggles. Soon, she returned to home and work.

Despite the progress, Chrissy felt like a robot, going through the motions. Driving to work, she didn't listen to the radio, but focused instead on counting the telephone poles. Her life was barren of emotion, with neither tears nor laughter. "I felt like I'd be on the medication for the rest of my life. I wasn't happy. I felt like my life was over, and I regretted having a child." Unable to dole out the love her son needed, she asked his daycare provider to shower him with maternal affection. Adding to her malaise was her husband's verbally and physically abusive behavior. She explains:

> My husband didn't handle it well. To this day, he says he failed me. Although I have forgiven him, I am still struggling with trusting him and feeling safe again, and he triggers a lot of my anxiety issues. We fell out of love with each other during the most difficult moments of my postpartum depression, and I am unsure if we will ever be able to fully recover from it emotionally. We are still trying to figure that out.

At her lowest, she grew suicidal. One day after taking her son to daycare, she returned home and fetched a firearm rather than going to work like she normally would. She drove around with it for 2 hours, trying to find a spot where she could go to end her life. Her boss called her cell phone repeatedly, sensing something wasn't right, and eventually her husband followed suit. "My husband called me, and a photo of him and my son popped up [in caller ID]. That phone call saved my life," she says. Though she didn't answer, it prompted her to return home and put away the weapon, without telling her husband what she'd been planning to do.

Chrissy's work as a principal financial analyst was a life raft: "My supervisor told me I was doing my job better than before [my sickness]. I held onto my job as the one thing that kept me going." Still, she struggled to focus at work, and she fought the urge to pace:

I would try to read a word or a sentence over and over, unable to string the letters and words together, unable to make sense of them. I appeared competent. No one could see that I, a well-educated and articulate former professional woman, could not read a sentence.

One day, something changed. "I walked out of work on a bright, sunny day in May 2014 and looked up at the sky. I said, 'God, give me the strength. I want to be the mom I never had,'" she says. "I turned the radio on in my car, and for the first time I was happy to pick up my son, and I didn't count telephone poles."

That was a turning point.

Recognizing she needed a change, she relocated to her hometown in southern Maryland, to be closer to her family and longtime friends. She has a new job, and she's seeing a therapist who specializes in women's mental health. She no longer takes anxiety or sleeping medications. Some hurdles remain, though. At times, she still battles symptoms of postpartum PTSD, often triggered by interactions with her husband. Rather than move with her, he opted to stay in Pennsylvania, so they spend weekends together and share their son bi-weekly. The time apart is helping her regroup.

As part of her healing, Chrissy hopes to pursue things she loves outside of motherhood, such as poetry, bowling, skiing, and piano lessons. She also wants to continue to raise awareness for perinatal mood disorders by sharing her story, and educating and encouraging other women. "Listen to your body. Keep talking. Don't be embarrassed, and keep going until you find the right person to help you," she advises mothers struggling after childbirth.

Postpartum depression is not a new thing. New moms have been suffering for years. It's just that, finally, people are talking about it.

It's also important to remember that PPD doesn't necessarily happen with the first child, nor does it plague a woman every time she has a child. If a woman knows her risk factors—such as past trauma or thyroid disease, for example—she can share them with her doctor, and together they can manage them. This way, if postpartum depression arises, it doesn't become unmanageable, she says: "The main thing is, talk. So many new moms just live in silence, too embarrassed to talk, and somehow we have to get through that it's OK. It's just a disease."

Though she still feels guilty for being unable to nurture her son during the first few months of his life, she is a better person for this experience. Chrissy says,

> I would not wish severe depression on anyone. However, looking back, I am now grateful for mine, and would not have it any other way. After all, not many people get to experience what the true meaning of life really is. I am blessed to have had that reality check.

Treating Postpartum PTSD

Experts agree that compared to postpartum depression, PTSD after childbirth has received less attention, including research on treatment. We do know that if it isn't addressed early, treatment might not be as successful, and could result in "significant psychological, social, and economic costs" (Beck et al., 2011, p. 226).

Among the types of therapy used to treat postpartum PTSD are:

▸ **Eye Movement Desensitization and Reprocessing** (EMDR) uses bilateral stimulation, such as a patient's eye movements, to help target and process disturbing memories and feelings.

▶ **Cognitive-Behavioral Therapy** (CBT) focuses on a patient's distorted, unhealthy thoughts and seeks to help her modify them and their resulting behaviors, thereby changing her mood and emotions for the better (for more on this, see Chapter 4).

▶ **Exposure Therapy** helps a patient repeatedly confront a source of trauma and, if possible, eliminate it as a source of distress.

Davis says other therapies are used, but they've not been researched for their effectiveness. "As with most psychotherapies, the general rule of thumb is that there is no therapy better than another," she says. The form of therapy must match the patient. For instance, some people prefer a verbal approach, while others respond well to body-centered therapies. She says,

> But most important to me is that the therapist has to be well-trained, and skilled in understanding not just the technique, but what might be needed to make sure the client is ready for the technique, to prepare for the technique. My favorite therapists are those that take their time, so that the client is not in danger of being re-traumatized.

An important part of treating postpartum PTSD lies in understanding that a woman has experienced a loss, and she's wading through grief over that loss, according to Barnes. "There's something unexpected and unplanned that didn't fit into the scheme of how she visualized her birth," she says. A therapist must help a mother make sense of the trauma and loss—otherwise, she won't fully heal.

Phyllis Klaus,[8] a California-based psychotherapist and social worker, takes this tack, and seeks first to learn her patients'

---

8   My personal communication with Phyllis Klaus took place between October 26, 2015, and October 25, 2016.

stories and build relationships with them. Rather than trying to fit someone into a category, Klaus uses a variety of skills to learn the specifics of a traumatic story. "I first help a client feel stabilized and grounded, and there are a lot of methods to do that. You have to realize when a person comes to see you, they're already in a vulnerable stage," says Klaus. She has spent more than 30 years specializing in perinatal mood and anxiety disorders, and is one of the founders of Prevention and Treatment of Traumatic Childbirth (PATTCh), a collective of birth and mental-health experts dedicated to preventing and treating traumatic childbirth. To help patients relax, Klaus might have them focus on slowing the rhythm of their breathing, or even smell roses or blow bubbles.

EMDR in Action

Klaus selects the form of therapy based on a patient's needs. EMDR is one she often uses to treat those with birth-related trauma and postpartum PTSD. But a patient doesn't have to be a new mother to benefit: it can help heal people of all ages with unresolved issues. "I use EMDR for many, many things. It's really powerful." It tends to be very effective, and regularly shows results in a short amount of time.

After a patient relaxes, Klaus works with her or him to develop something called "internal resources." These are images of calm, safe places, or of protectors, such as heroines or angels: "Whatever works that gives you a sense of feeling loved, nurtured, and supported." Klaus reinforces the images with a form of bilateral stimulation—for example, through eye movement, or by tapping back and forth, on the left and right sides of the patient's body: "That's very, very helpful for people. You begin to integrate those resources, so when you do the trauma work they feel more supported internally. It's like an inner guide or protector, and it feels safer to do the work."

At this point, Klaus asks a patient to visualize and explain her traumatic story. In some cases, it's necessary to do this several times. They work together to determine the emotions a patient still harbors related to the trauma, such as anger, fear, powerlessness, or betrayal, as well as the negative beliefs. An example of a negative belief is when someone thinks her needs aren't important, or that she has no power. Klaus helps a patient figure out where in her body she's holding the tension associated with her negative beliefs and emotions.

After that, Klaus helps the patient develop a set of positive beliefs, such as, "I have the right to be heard. My needs and choices are important. I had no choice at the time, but I can create new choices now." She again uses bilateral stimulation, reinforcing the positive beliefs.

EMDR allows a person to physically and mentally release negative beliefs and emotions about a trauma, and replace them with positive beliefs. Bilateral stimulation is key to this process, Klaus says, and what differentiates it from other forms of therapy.

It's important to not just address the trauma itself, but to go further, and work to heal the unfinished business left behind. Many women feel their bodies failed them, for instance, so they need affirmation that their bodies did the best they could. A woman can use this validation to strengthen herself. She might even use the knowledge she acquires through therapy as she plans for a future birth. Trauma holds a person back from something that needed to happen, Klaus says, "and if you can help it happen, then you can heal."

When it comes to medication, Jennifer Zimmerman,[9] cofounder of the group Solace for Mothers: Healing After Traumatic Childbirth, says it "does not seem to do anything to heal trauma, although it can provide relief of certain symptoms, so in some cases it may

---

9   My personal communication with Jennifer Zimmerman took place between October 22, 2015, and December 8, 2015.

be a beneficial tool in conjunction with therapy. It should just be understood that it won't be a cure on its own."

Some forms of medication have been found effective in helping treat PTSD in the general population, particularly antidepressants, according to Dekel's review of the literature. If these medications are safe during pregnancy and for postpartum women who are breastfeeding, they can be used to treat postpartum PTSD, according to Dekel.

> There needs to be more studies on the long-term effects of the use of antidepressants during the postpartum period. Antidepressants may be effective for some women, but not all. In some cases, antidepressants need to be combined with psychological treatment. We are still far from personal medicine in which treatment is tailored towards the specific needs of each patient.

Postpartum PTSD Q&A With Jennifer Zimmerman

Cofounder, Solace for Mothers: Healing After Traumatic Childbirth, http://www.solaceformothers.org/

KC: **Based on your work, what have you seen in terms of the forms of treatment that are best for those diagnosed with postpartum PTSD?**

JZ: I don't feel I can say any particular therapy is best, because so many women find healing in so many different ways. As far as standard therapeutic treatments, most of the women on Solace for Mothers who have tried EMDR therapy report that it is effective and helpful in their healing. CBT or other forms of therapy can also be very useful for some women. I have never heard of anyone trying exposure therapy for birth trauma. ... Creative expression seems to be something many women find helpful. Things such as writing, artwork, music, or dance can be very healing. Bodywork is also really helpful. Many types of alternative therapies are popular as well. The online peer-support forum we have set up on our website has also been very beneficial for many women.

KC: **Some experts say postpartum PTSD is a new area of scientific research, and understanding of the disorder is limited. Would you agree with this?**

JZ: I don't know that it's new. There has been a lot of research into this area and a lot of interesting findings about the maternity-care system, and how we treat new mothers and infants. However, it can take 15 to 20 years for clinical research to make it into standard practice. I think it has been hard for doctors and mental-health providers to accept that women could have been traumatized during what is considered a normal life experience. It is also hard to accept that their trauma may be the result of mistreatment by the health care providers they encountered while giving birth. It seems more like denial than a lack of research that limits understanding of this disorder.

KC: **Do you feel that women with postpartum PTSD are often misdiagnosed and receive the wrong treatment? Or perhaps they're treated for co-existing symptoms of postpartum depression, and the PTSD isn't fully addressed, prolonging their suffering?**

JZ: Yes, absolutely. Many women who I have encountered talk about how they were diagnosed with PPD and medicated, and then go on to tell me a long story of their birth trauma and how that was the start of their issues. What is very problematic is that a key feature of postpartum PTSD is avoidance of reminders of the trauma. At 6 weeks postpartum, new mothers are expected to visit the health care provider who likely played a key role in their traumatic experience. Not only that, but their private areas will be examined by this provider, putting them right back in the same position of vulnerability that they were in when they gave birth.

Women who have experienced birth trauma may avoid this visit, as well as some or all of the well-baby checks their baby should be scheduled for in the first couple years of life. But even if a woman goes to these doctor visits, and even if she is given the standard postpartum-depression assessment to fill out, her trauma still may not be recognized. She may not have identified what is happening to her as "trauma," so she will not be able to articulate that to her provider. If her provider is looking for depression, that is what her provider will find. Trauma is not currently assessed for, so trauma is not usually identified, even if it is the predominant issue women are dealing with.

Medication can relieve some symptoms, but the trauma won't heal until it is dealt with appropriately. If a woman feels she may have been misdiagnosed, she can search online for a PTSD self-assessment tool, and see if her symptoms match up with that. I would then suggest that she find a therapist who specifically works with trauma.

KC: How does Solace for Mothers help women who have postpartum PTSD? Can it also be a resource for those who might be dealing with, say, a traumatic birth, and experiencing symptoms of postpartum anxiety or depression, but they don't have symptoms of postpartum PTSD?

JZ: Solace for Mothers helps women who have experienced a traumatic birth, whether or not they qualify for the diagnosis of PTSD. Some women may not have all of the components of diagnosable PTSD, but are still dealing with significant trauma-based symptoms. Linked from our website is an online support group for women who experienced birth trauma. This group is private and is not searchable by Google, and we ask that only women who themselves experienced birth trauma join. We also provide a directory of mental-health care providers who identify as working with women with birth-trauma issues. It can be difficult for many women with birth trauma to find a therapist who understands that giving birth can, in some cases, be a traumatic experience, which led us to developing this directory.

Katie's Story

Some women, like Katie Kmiecik,[10] are so moved by their postpartum experiences, they tailor their careers. Katie, who had been a therapist before her daughter was born in March 2011, decided to specialize in PMADs after she experienced PPD, PPA, postpartum OCD, and postpartum PTSD.

The baby was born via C-section, and spent a week in the neonatal intensive care unit (NICU). "As soon as the baby was out, I looked at her and had zero connection to her," says Katie, co-founder of the Postpartum Wellness Center in Hoffman Estates, Illinois. "I said she was cute, because I knew I was supposed to say something, and a wave of anxiety overcame me."

Her daughter's stay in the NICU exacerbated Katie's anxiety, and she later developed symptoms of postpartum PTSD. She avoided reminders of the NICU and the hospital. Though her doctor said she needed a dilation and curettage (D&C) to stanch her postpartum bleeding, she didn't get the procedure for 10 months, due to extreme dread of returning to the hospital. "I just kept putting it off because I couldn't go, and hospitals, to me, were the worst thing that ever happened. I didn't want to go back in there."

Katie was hypervigilant. Any sign of irregularity with the baby, and she pegged it as an emergency. At one point, she called 911, fearing the child wasn't breathing. As it turned out, she was just sleeping soundly. Another of her symptoms was an exaggerated startle response: "I was scared to death of everything, just waiting for the next shoe to drop. Like veterans [who] jump when they hear a bang." Sensations she associated with the NICU also bothered her, such as a beep triggering memories of the baby monitors there. "I was always on high alert. It was exhausting and constant."

---

10 My personal communication with Katie Kmiecik took place between September 4, 2015, and March 4, 2016.

Meanwhile, she experienced symptoms of other PMADs (see Chapter 4), and after 6 months, she finally shared her agony with a close friend. The same day she sought professional help. She ended up seeing two therapists and one psychiatrist—all in different practices—and she was prescribed Zoloft and Wellbutrin for the depression and anxiety. One therapist used cognitive-behavioral therapy to treat her postpartum anxiety and OCD. The other addressed her postpartum PTSD with EMDR, and it started working during the first session.

According to the EMDR Institute,

> Repeated studies show that by using EMDR therapy people can experience the benefits of psychotherapy that once took years to make a difference. It is widely assumed that severe emotional pain requires a long time to heal. EMDR therapy shows that the mind can in fact heal from psychological trauma much as the body recovers from physical trauma. When you cut your hand, your body works to close the wound. If a foreign object or repeated injury irritates the wound, it festers and causes pain. Once the block is removed, healing resumes. EMDR therapy demonstrates that a similar sequence of events occurs with mental processes. The brain's information processing system naturally moves toward mental health. If the system is blocked or imbalanced by the impact of a disturbing event, the emotional wound festers and can cause intense suffering. Once the block is removed, healing resumes (n.d.).

As evidence of how well EMDR worked for her, Katie points to the fact that since therapy, she's returned to the NICU, and she isn't bothered by the sights and sounds there. She now gears her work toward helping mothers with babies in intensive care.

She credits the combination of medication and therapy with helping her heal. "I'm a big fan of medications. They can really get you through. You're hurting yourself by not trying the medication," she says. She points out that if a perinatal mood disorder is spurred by chemical imbalance, that won't be recalibrated without medicine.

By the time her daughter was one, Katie felt much better, but still worked hard at rebuilding. Once her daughter was two, she was 95 percent recovered. As for why she waited 6 months to get help, she was embarrassed and afraid, and chalked up her trouble to being weak—a bad mother and a bad person. Postpartum mood disorders don't come up in regular conversation. But she's working to change that. In 2013, she and her partners launched the Postpartum Wellness Center, which specializes in helping women and families affected by perinatal mood and anxiety disorders. It has been a fast-growing endeavor, and Katie finds herself busier than she ever imagined she would be.

What Trauma Taught Me

Trauma can be a great teacher. Once I gained distance on the difficult events surrounding Noah's birth, I wanted to learn from them. I also wanted to prevent a recurrence, because we planned to have another child.

First I considered how my attitudes and behaviors might have been stumbling blocks:

▸ believing others knew best, and not trusting my own instincts;

▸ wanting to be cooperative;

▸ not speaking up about my fears and concerns; and

▸ not asking enough questions.

The second time around, I would change my approach. I would trust my instincts, speak up, ask questions, and be my own best advocate. By doing so, I would have a shot at a better birth experience—or at least I would be empowered by applying what I had learned.

The next thing I did was to find a new OB practice and hospital. We had moved out of the city by the time we were ready for the next baby, so this part was easy. I would've switched caregivers, even if we hadn't moved, because I knew change on every level was essential to achieving a different experience. Once I was pregnant again, I shared the trauma of Noah's birth with doctors and nurses in my new OB practice. I explained what I wanted to avoid this time. I made sure my history was recorded in my chart. Most importantly, an early induction was out of the question, unless it was a life-or-death matter for the baby or me. By the time I was 9 months pregnant, everyone knew my story, and they agreed to work with me.

A few weeks before my second birth, I toured the maternity ward of our new hospital. I left in tears. What if more trauma awaited me, despite everything I was doing? I knew it was unlikely that this baby would come into the world the same way Noah had. Emotionally, however, something was missing. I had to confront what I considered to be my abuser: the Chicago hospital where Noah was born. I needed to tell someone official there about what had happened. I needed someone to apologize. So I called the hospital.

I reached a nurse, and shared with her my concerns about some of the hospital's practices—encouraging an induction ahead of a due date, and my early discharge. Receptive and apologetic, she assured me that it was standard back then to schedule inductions before a child was due, even if it wasn't a medical necessity. That standard had changed, she said, because they saw too many inductions ending in trauma. She wished me the best with my daughter.

Talking to her made me feel better. I was heartened to hear they had halted early inductions, and I felt less alone—other women at that hospital had faced the same situation. The phone call didn't erase the past trauma. But relaying my story, even after more than 2 years, brought a measure of mental relief and empowerment. It gave me hope as I faced childbirth again. It was a necessary step, and it helped.

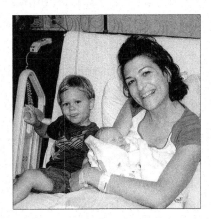

First encounters: Noah meets his sister, Syma, on the day she was born, August 28, 2011, in Naperville, Illinois.

When I went into labor with my second child—my daughter, Syma—the first thing I did on arriving at the hospital was recount my past to the nurses and doctors: I had a difficult first birth with complications and trauma, and I later battled postpartum depression. I made it clear that I had learned a lot, and I was determined to have a better experience. This was important. The doctor on-call when I arrived wasn't one of the OBs in my practice, and I couldn't assume anyone from my practice had communicated my desires to him—or to anyone else at the hospital. He and the nurses had excellent bedside manner, and they worked with me to achieve what I wanted. I lobbied hard against Pitocin. I never ended up needing it. Interestingly, among all the other women in labor and delivery that night, I was the only one *not* receiving Pitocin.

I made it without an epidural for around ten hours. Ultimately, I opted for one that subdued the contractions, but maintained feeling in my lower body. It also allowed me to sleep for several hours. I made this choice based on the epidural I had with Noah, which left my lower half entirely numb and made pushing difficult. It was a wise move that gave me what I needed and wanted during the birth: rest and sensation.

I awoke refreshed, and ready to deliver the baby. After only a few pushes, Syma was born.

This time, it wasn't as if I was watching the birth happen to someone else. It was happening to *me*, and I could feel it. The ethereal sensations weren't manufactured by pain medication. They came from the friction of my daughter's body against mine, as she moved from womb to world. When I reflect on that moment, I revel in it.

I had learned how to help myself through self-advocacy, so Syma's birth was a mental and physical victory. It was something I made happen because I acted on what I had learned with Noah. Most of all, I overcame problems from that first experience. My body wasn't an inferior maternal vehicle, after all. I *was* capable of achieving the type of childbirth I had imagined. It wasn't an independent achievement, though. I had help from others, especially from my care providers, skilled in both medicine and bedside manner.

I doubt Syma's birth would have seemed half as rich if I hadn't suffered my first time. It allowed me to appreciate something I otherwise would've taken for granted—a smooth delivery, birth, and postpartum. It led to knowledge, self-strength, and a different experience. The choices I made my second time were rooted in suffering the first time, and they allowed me to stay whole. I wasn't the fractured version of myself that I had been after Noah was born. Though it seems contradictory, it's true: suffering enriches our lives in ways nothing else can.

Still, it doesn't have a lot of selling points. Suffering conjures notions of losing control, and paves the way to a land of many fears. It's more comfortable to maintain control and not suffer. Cozy as it is, this is an illusion. Illness, whether mental or physical, wakes me from the dream and reminds me that I'm not in control of most things. This can spark a sense of loneliness—but it doesn't mean I'm alone. Someone is in control, who sees and knows my struggles and fights on my behalf: God. Knowing this brings comfort. It's not my job to control everything, and there's a quiet freedom in remembering that.

Coming to terms with all of this will take a lifetime, and along the way, I can squeeze good out of bad. Trauma wasn't the end of my childbirth story. It was a beginning, one that delivered a remarkable experience the second time.

My ability to move through PPD and find healing hasn't meant an end to all struggle, though. Motherhood is defined by detours and trials. As life continues to prove that, I pray that I gain strength as a mother, a woman, and ideally, as someone who helps others with what I've learned.

CHAPTER 3

Postpartum Depression and Anxiety

Worse Than We Think

Maybe you have to know the darkness

before you can appreciate the light.

MADELEINE L'ENGLE,

A Ring of Endless Light

After I cleared the first trimester of pregnancy, Matt and I drove to Ohio to share the news with my family. Sitting at my brother's kitchen table, I brimmed with excitement as Jim recounted stories from early parenthood. Looking at Matt, he said, "Watch Krissy after she has the baby. The postpartum-depression stuff is real, and it can just creep up on her."

I was surprised. My sister-in-law hadn't let on that she suffered after my nephews were born. But I didn't give it much thought. Postpartum depression wouldn't happen to me, I figured. I was a happy person with a can-do spirit.

The only other PPD mention I heard while pregnant was from a nurse leading my new-parenting class. She said mothers might have unusual feelings of sadness after childbirth, or may not want to leave the baby's side for fear of something bad happening. In these cases, she suggested calling a health care provider.

In hindsight, I was unwarned about how serious perinatal mood and anxiety disorders are. After I had Noah, my OB told me she hadn't made it an issue because I wasn't a likely candidate. I didn't have a personal or family history of depression, I wasn't facing marital or financial stress, and I had plenty of supportive friends and family. Still, I wish someone had talked to me. Other parents I spoke with felt the same.

Depression Casts a Wide Net

Ashley,[11] a mother of two, had postpartum depression after the birth of her first child in 2007. She feels someone should have cautioned her ahead of time. "You read all the books to prepare, and you have the baby, and it's nothing like the book said. I was trying my best to be prepared, and I have never felt so unprepared

[11] Ashley's real name has been changed to protect her privacy.

in my life," says Ashley, an attorney. "No one had ever talked to me about life with a newborn being difficult, and as a result, I hid my depression as best I could from everyone around me ... until it consumed me."

Like many, Ashley concealed her suffering. Mental-health problems are laden with a stigma so powerful, it often silences people. New mothers who say they were afraid to speak up point to worries of being sent to a mental-health facility, someone taking their child, or their husband or partner abandoning them. They believe they are the only ones who have ever plummeted to such treacherous depths.

But they are hardly alone. PPD is more prevalent than many of us realize. I certainly wasn't aware of its wide reach before I began research on this book. Depending on the population studied and how depression is defined, the incidence of postpartum depression varies. Typically, the range is between 12 and 25 percent of new mothers. In some high-risk groups, rates are as steep as 40 percent or more (Kendall-Tackett, 2016). During pregnancy, between 14 and 23 percent of women will battle symptoms of depression (American College of Obstetricians and Gynecologists, 2009).

A UK-based study published in 2010 found that depression among mothers and fathers was highest in the first year after childbirth. By the time the child reached 12 years of age, 39 percent of mothers and 21 percent of fathers had faced depression (Davé et al.).

In 2013, the study results of the largest depression screening of postpartum women so far showed that 14 percent of new mothers screened positive for postpartum depression (Wisner et al.). "It's a huge public health problem. A woman's mental health has a profound effect on fetal development as well as her child's physical and emotional development," said lead study author Dr. Katherine L. Wisner (Paul, 2013). Wisner is the director of Northwestern University's Asher Center for the Study and

Treatment of Depressive Disorders, and a professor of psychiatry and obstetrics at Northwestern's Feinberg School of Medicine.

After Wisner's study was released, postpartum blogger and activist Katherine Stone[12] wrote that a lot of the media had reacted to the 14 percent figure as surprising: "I'm sure this makes all of you snicker, given that it's not surprising AT ALL (yes, I'm yelling) to anyone who has spent any time either suffering from postpartum depression or working with moms who do" (Stone, 2013). Stone, who had postpartum depression and OCD after the birth of her first child (Becoming Fierce and Powerful, n.d.), says the number of women who encounter PPD is closer to 20 percent.

> *No one had ever talked to me about life with a newborn being difficult, and as a result, I hid my depression as best I could from everyone around me ... until it consumed me.*
>
> Ashley, a mother of two who had postpartum depression and anxiety

Like Ashley, I was startled by trials after childbirth. The shower was the first place I cried, because it was my only private haven. We lived in a high-rise apartment, my mother-in-law was in town, and the baby was rarely more than a few feet from me. At first I thought the tears would be fleeting. I feared my mother-in-law would think I was incapable of being a mother. She had four children and had served as an American-born missionary in France while she raised them. I couldn't even get it right in my home country. The threat of frightening my husband, or losing his trust, was worst of all.

After a few nights of crying in the shower, I knew something was wrong. Hiding sapped my energy, so I wept in front of my husband and his mother, shared my fears, and reached out for help.

---

12   My personal communication with Katherine Stone took place between March 4, 2011, and April 1, 2011.

Baby Blues

Initially, my close friends and family speculated that I might have the baby blues, which strike up to 80 percent of all new mothers. Many confuse the blues with postpartum depression, but they're not the same thing.

In the first days or weeks postpartum, four out of five mothers feel sad, frustrated, tearful, anxious, and/or overwhelmed, what many women call "an emotional roller-coaster," says Dr. Christina Hibbert.[13] Too many families aren't made aware of this reality, according to Hibbert, an Arizona-based clinical psychologist and expert on maternal mental health, grief, and loss. Dads can have the blues, too, and are more prone to them if their partners have symptoms (Hibbert, 2012). Hibbert herself grappled with perinatal mood disorders after the births of each of her four children. She writes,

> If you think about it, it makes perfect sense that your emotions might be a little out of whack after pregnancy and childbirth, considering all your body and mind have been through. The abrupt changes in hormones, sleep deprivation, and the psychological adjustment to becoming a parent, not to mention the exhaustion of labor and delivery, can easily trigger fluctuations in emotions (Hibbert, 2012).

The blues aren't an illness. They're a temporary, "normal reaction to the stress surrounding childbirth," according to Hibbert, and they usually fade within 2 weeks (Hibbert, 2012). Mothers might incorrectly believe their PPD is simply a case of the blues, and fail to seek treatment. Hibbert says,

---

13 My personal communication with Dr. Christina Hibbert took place between December 11, 2013, and May 30, 2014.

Even providers often diagnose women with "The Baby Blues" when they really have PPD. The marker is about two weeks, or symptoms that intensify over time. So, if a mom is still struggling with [the blues] a month out, even if her symptoms aren't very intense, she's more likely dealing with mild PPD. ... Because of this, many women do not seek help, believing it will just "get better" with time. Sometimes, it does. Many times, it does not.

My symptoms persisted past 2 weeks and were more intense than the blues, which meant I had something more serious—a full-blown perinatal mood and anxiety disorder.

Prenatal and Postpartum Depression

Ashley's Story

In the week after her son was born, Ashley found herself crying frequently in the shower, and worrying that she wasn't fit to be a mother and wife. "I thought about leaving them, that they would be better off without me. I struggled with breastfeeding, too, so I felt like a complete failure," she says. Her depression led to severe insomnia, so even the smallest setbacks seemed monumental.

A sense of worthlessness defined her days, and she shared with her husband that she didn't feel right. He assumed she was distraught because of breastfeeding. Ashley says,

Despite his best intention, I think he was completely confused. I desperately needed help, but we both just thought I had the baby blues and it would pass. He had no idea how to help me, and I think it scared him. Neither of us were informed about PPD until I was diagnosed.

She attended a mothers' group led by a social worker, and it proved to be a saving grace. "I couldn't relax. I could not sleep for the life of me. One day, I just broke down at the group session and was crying." The social worker pulled her aside, suggested she might have postpartum depression, and encouraged her to seek treatment.

When the baby was 4 months old, she started seeing a psychiatrist, who prescribed Zoloft and sleeping pills. The sleeping medication helped her regain consistent sleep, and that in turn reduced the anxiety. She also went to talk-therapy sessions once a week, with a psychologist. Ashley felt much better when she went back to work, 6 months after the baby was born. She now wishes she had sought treatment sooner.

Ashley had a combination of postpartum depression and anxiety, which is often the case. Northwestern's Wisner says, "Clinicians need to know that the most common clinical presentation in the post-birth period is more complex than a single episode of depression. The depression is recurrent and superimposed on an anxiety disorder" (Paul, 2013).

Symptoms

Symptoms can surface at any point during pregnancy, or up to a year after the baby is born. Women might experience anger, irritability, a lack of interest in the baby, or an inability to eat or sleep. They could feel guilt, shame, or hopelessness, accompanied by crying and sadness. Losing interest in things they once enjoyed is common. Thoughts of hurting themselves or the baby are perhaps the worst of the symptoms (Postpartum Support International, n.d.).

Risk Factors

Predicting depression is a challenge. "We don't know why one woman gets it and another doesn't. ... We know there are all these different factors intermingling, but we don't know why there is a perfect storm," says Karen Kleiman, founder of The Postpartum Stress Center.

Still, experts agree that risk factors exist. Among some of them are:

Clinicians need to know that the most common clinical presentation in the post-birth period is more complex than a single episode of depression. The depression is recurrent and superimposed on an anxiety disorder.

Dr. Katherine L. Wisner, director of Northwestern University's Asher Center for the Study and Treatment of Depressive Disorders

▶ a past episode of postpartum depression;

▶ depression or anxiety during pregnancy;

▶ a history of depression or bipolar disorder prior to pregnancy;

▶ a history of anxiety disorder;

▶ prior physical or sexual abuse;

▶ a lack of social support;

▶ premenstrual dysphoric disorder (PMDD or PMS);

▶ financial or marital stress;

▶ complications during pregnancy or childbirth;

▶ a recent, major event, such as the death of a loved one, losing a job or moving to a new home;

▶ giving birth to multiples;

▶ an infant in neonatal intensive care (NICU);

▶ infertility treatments;

▶ thyroid imbalance; and

▶ any form of diabetes, including type 1, type 2, or gestational (Nonacs, 2007; Postpartum Support International, n.d.).

Prenatal and Postpartum Anxiety

Leah's Story

Leah,[14] a teacher and mother of two, developed anxiety, depression, and PTSD after her first child was born with a heart defect in 2010. The morning after her son arrived, she attended a new mothers' orientation, and returned to find her baby gone. Doctors had whisked him away, and told her he was turning blue while they observed him.

"The first time I saw him, he was already sedated, hooked up to tubes, in an incubator. I just came into the nursery and they were trying to explain it to me ... it was just like a nightmare," Leah says. Her son was transferred to a different hospital, where a pediatric cardiologist performed a procedure to widen one of his heart valves.

Meanwhile, she feared she was to blame for the flaw in her baby's heart: "This was my body. Did I do something wrong, to cause a problem? I tried to be so careful during my pregnancy." She fixated on the one sip of champagne she took during a New Year's celebration, thinking it could've been the root of her son's trouble. Doctors never told her she *didn't* cause the defect, and to this day, she wonders if it was her fault.

Dr. Linda R. Chambliss,[15] director of the division of maternal fetal medicine at St. Joseph's Hospital and Medical Center in Phoenix, says a mother's sip of champagne wouldn't trigger a baby's congenital heart defect. But other things can increase a woman's risks, including uncontrolled conditions like diabetes or a deficiency in folic acid.

When Leah's son came home at about eleven days old, he needed shots for several weeks—something she didn't feel

---

14   Leah's real name has been changed to protect her privacy.
15   My personal communication with Dr. Linda R. Chambliss took place between June 13, 2014, and July 27, 2014.

comfortable doing, and another source of stress. She also had difficulty nursing.

Her anxiety became more noticeable when the baby was a few months old. She felt overwhelmed, plagued by racing thoughts and trouble sleeping. To release energy surging through her body, she would shake her hands, arms, and legs, and she would pace in the middle of the night. "I didn't know what to do. I was in a crazy, frantic mindset where I didn't know what to do with my body." Tremendous anger sent her on yelling and throwing sprees. "I felt like smashing things. I remember taking these Duplo blocks—I threw them down the hallway out of madness and anger and rage."

Prevalence, Symptoms, and Risk Factors

Leah's racing thoughts, sleep disturbances, and inability to sit still were symptoms of postpartum anxiety. Others include constant worry, feeling something bad will happen, trouble eating, dizziness, hot flashes, and nausea. About 6 percent of pregnant women and 10 percent of postpartum women develop anxiety. Risk factors include a personal or family history of anxiety, previous perinatal depression or anxiety, and thyroid imbalance (Postpartum Support International, n.d.).

In addition to general anxiety, there are specific anxiety disorders, including postpartum obsessive-compulsive disorder (PPOCD) and postpartum panic disorder. Postpartum OCD, the focus of Chapter 4, is a combination of intrusive thoughts and repetitive behaviors. Postpartum panic disorder is characterized by recurring panic attacks and nervousness. A panic attack might involve shortness of breath, chest pain, claustrophobia, dizziness, heart palpitations, and numbness and tingling in the extremities (Postpartum Support International, n.d.).

Seeking Treatment

Long bouts of crying and intrusive images were the two major symptoms of my experience with postpartum depression. I tolerated them on my own for only a short while. I knew that by sharing my burden, I could lighten my load. So I sought informal talk therapy with family and close friends. While I saw some relief, it wasn't the cure I needed. I didn't want to wait any longer. I had no experience in this arena, and I couldn't be sure I would get better on my own. After a few weeks, I called my OB for help. Patience isn't one of my strong suits; in this instance, that was a boon. I believe I rebounded swiftly because I acted quickly.

Deciding if and when to seek professional help can be tricky, and it's unique to the individual. Kleiman and Dr. Valerie Davis Raskin's book, *This Isn't What I Expected: Overcoming Postpartum Depression* (2013), is a resource that can help you determine a plan of action. The authors outline a five-step recovery plan that encourages women first to use their internal resources as support, a move that alleviates symptoms in mild cases. When PPD is more intense, women must consider professional help. They explain:

> Most women put off seeking professional help until they have tried to get better on their own. Some women, especially those who have been treated by a mental-health professional in the past, immediately turn to a therapist as the first step (Kleiman & Raskin, 2013, p. 27).

Kleiman and Raskin encourage women to be receptive to all available resources to help them recover, such as their husbands, extended families, family doctors, psychiatrists, therapists, medication, new-mothers' groups at a church or synagogue, and local PPD self-help groups. The book provides information on therapy and medication, and the various facets to consider with each. As the authors point out, "Medication is not the only treatment for PPD and is generally most helpful when combined with therapy" (2013, p. 107). They outline the different reasons women hesitate when it comes to medication, and offer reassurances. Not all women with PPD need medication. Treatment is based on severity of symptoms, patient preferences, her responses to other treatments or changes in support, and the risk of side effects. Some women pursue only therapy. Others are only interested in medication. Kleiman and Raskin write:

> Certain symptoms, such as loss of concentration, severe insomnia, confusion, extreme indecisiveness, suicidal thoughts, and severe feelings of guilt make it nearly impossible to work in therapy. Medication can stabilize these symptoms enough to allow you to invest the psychological energy that therapy requires. We strongly believe that in severe cases of PPD, medication contributes to a quicker, fuller, longer-lasting recovery (2013, p. 109).

With therapy, the goal should be helping a woman find relief from her symptoms and return to the level at which she previously functioned. Effective short-term therapies include:

▸ **Supportive therapy:** Conversation-based; uses praise, advice, clarification, confrontation, and interpretation to help a patient gain understanding.

▸ **Cognitive-behavioral therapy:** Focuses on a patient's distorted thoughts that reinforce her depression, and seeks to help her modify the thoughts, thereby changing her mood and emotions.

▸ **Interpersonal psychotherapy:** Focuses on problems in key relationships, and how the relationships affect a patient's ability to function.

▸ **Brief dynamic therapy:** Centers on the importance of early childhood relationships and experiences, and how they relate to the patient as an adult, especially during her mood disorder.

▸ **Group therapy:** Group sessions are either professional, and led by a trained therapist, or peer-led by other postpartum women who share their experiences. Groups can be focused on specific topics and time-limited, or open-ended and unstructured (Kleiman & Raskin, 2013, pp. 156-159).

Dr. Christina Hibbert, who founded the Arizona Postpartum Wellness Coalition, a nonprofit that educates women, families, and providers on perinatal mental health, says the agents of recovery that seem to work best for most people are support groups or therapy. "Most of these moms really need to share what they have been through and want to talk about it," Hibbert says. Therapy provides new coping skills. As a psychologist, Hibbert strives to give her patients tools to help them flourish in life. "That is what you can learn from therapy, from someone you like and trust." If therapy alone doesn't work, she encourages women to try adding medication. In severe cases, it is critical. "Sometimes therapy doesn't really work until the meds kick in. Therapy and medicine are the gold standard for moderate-to-severe PPD," she says.

The medical records from my OB's office show that I was diagnosed with severe postpartum depression. In the thick of it, I would've agreed. Now, with more than 7 years of perspective, and after interviewing women for this book and talking with others anecdotally, I characterize my experience as moderate. I received the gold standard in treatment, a combination of medication and therapy, and I'll always be grateful for it.

Still, it wasn't the diagnosis that drove me to write this book. It was the number of postpartum stories I encountered once I shared my own experience. Dr. Diana L. Barnes, a psychotherapist who specializes in women's reproductive mental health, says a woman's personal story should take precedence over her diagnosis: "The bottom line is, what is the woman's story that's leading to the way she feels? What we call it is really secondary." While it's important to name and diagnose a patient's illness, that's only part of her job as a therapist. "Every woman has a story, and if I understand the story, then she's going to get better. If all I do is treat the symptoms, she might get better, but there won't be the larger sense of change."

What's Left Unsaid: Self-Blame and Feeling Like a Failure

Some symptoms of mood and anxiety disorders don't make the clinically recognized lists, things like self-blame and feeling like a failure. But they're no less real.

Chambliss says they can be contributors to and symptoms of PMADs. "Women are very quick to blame themselves when something goes wrong. You see it all the time," she says. This can be fuel for depression, and once the depression is there, a woman may get stuck in a vicious loop of self-flagellating.

In my case these, feelings appeared within a week of Noah's arrival. I saw myself failing during childbirth, when doctors resorted to forceps and I tore, and later, when I had complications from the tear and ended up in the ER. Despite friends and family assuring me these were circumstances beyond my control, I still condemned myself. Hadn't I caused all of this by inducing early? Only a bad mother would oust her baby from her womb. Such dark thoughts fueled my illness, and as the depression deepened, they persisted.

Leah confronted similar feelings. A tremendous burden of failure fell upon her one day as she administered her son's shots:

> [W]hen I messed one up and didn't insert the needle
> correctly and my son screamed and cried, that's
> when I felt like a failure ... I just sobbed and sobbed
> because I didn't want to do the shots in the first place,
> and there I was alone, and messing up and hurting
> my child because I didn't do it right.

She was ensnared in an unrelenting cycle of perceived failures: wondering if she had bungled the pregnancy and caused her child to be born with a heart defect, trouble with nursing, and then struggling with his shots. "I would hit the bed with my fist and I would say, 'I'm a failure,'—yell it, like, 20 times—and this rage overtook me to the point where my husband said, 'I can't handle this.'" They moved in with her parents for a short time, to get more support.

Eventually, Leah found a therapist who practiced EMDR, a form of therapy geared to helping a patient physically and mentally release negative beliefs and emotions about a trauma, and replace them with positive beliefs. (For more on EMDR, see Chapter 2.) Leah calls her EMDR therapy "amazing." Within a few months of starting, she was able to sleep through the night again. She also had a breakthrough. Her therapist helped her revisit and heal from a traumatic experience she had before giving birth. During time she spent at a children's home in Africa, Leah tried to resuscitate a little girl found submerged in a washbasin. Leah wasn't able to revive the child, and she didn't process the horror of the situation and its impact on her. "But it was very raw, and I felt like a failure. It was very traumatic to be in the spotlight and doing CPR. It was a very awful experience. I had never dealt with it."

EMDR helped her address the guilt she had related to the girl drowning. She says,

> [T]he idea is that the trauma of my son's near-death
> experience "landed" on ... that unprocessed trauma

in Africa years earlier. Even though her drowning was not my fault, I still felt like I failed at reviving her to life with CPR. With EMDR, my therapist helped me see my strength in putting myself in a position to help the child, even though she was probably already dead and there was nothing that could be done.

Reflecting on her postpartum trials, Leah doesn't see herself as a failure. She realizes she was strong, because she didn't give up, despite feeling overwhelmed and out of control: "Though I completely fell apart, I took very good care of my son through it all. That, to me, is amazing."

Women with perfectionist tendencies may grapple more with the sense of failure than others. Ashley, who calls herself a "Type A" personality, saw a series of blunders that started when she went into labor in the 26th week of her pregnancy. For 10 weeks, she was on strict bed rest with a Terbutaline pump in her leg, giving her medicine to prevent preterm labor.

"So I was isolated through the part of my pregnancy where I should have been showing and celebrating with others, including the holiday season," she says. Her baby was born at 36 weeks, after delivery with the help of a vacuum, which is a cup with a handle, and a pump that attaches to a baby's head and guides it out of the birth canal (Mayo Clinic Staff, 2015).

Then she had difficulty nursing. "I think I expected breastfeeding to come easily, and when it didn't, it led to feelings of inadequacy that compounded my depression," Ashley says. No one and nothing—including the variety of literature she read on having a child—warned her about potential postpartum perils. It all left her feeling as if she couldn't meet any of her own expectations.

I am a well-educated, professional person. You read all the books to prepare, and [then] you have the baby, and it's nothing like the book said. I was trying my best to be prepared, and I have never felt so unprepared in my life.

Part of why we feel we have failed is because the reality of new motherhood lies in stark contrast to our ideal picture of it. Barnes refers to this as a mythology about what new mothers are supposed to feel, think, look like, and say. "If you find your experience doesn't fit into the cultural mythology, it can feel very shaming. That in itself can lead to a downward spiral of depression," says Barnes, who treats women and their families at The Center for Postpartum Health in California.

What creates the mythology? We idealize mothers. That's the good and bad news. The bad news is that we don't leave any room for the real experience of motherhood. You can love your children, but still find new motherhood unbelievably exhausting and overwhelming. We don't see the distinction.

Unfortunately for some of us, postpartum depression is part of motherhood. Coming to terms with this, and accepting that it's okay to *not* be okay—even when you're a new mother—is essential to fighting mood disorders. This acceptance will also strengthen us for one of the roughest parts of the fight: stigma. It is a behemoth for everyone who struggles with their mental health—women and men, young and not-as-young, and those with temporary or longer-term illnesses. I touch on stigma throughout the book, and focus on it in Chapter 6.

CHAPTER 4

Over and Over

The Unsettling Spiral of Postpartum OCD

As for me, I call to God,
and the Lord saves me.
Evening, morning, and noon,
I cry out in distress,
and he hears my voice.

Psalm 55:16-17, New International

Version (NIV)

The week after I had Noah, my physical wounds started to settle. I was eager to trade calamity for calm. What was I thinking? This was motherhood, after all. A fresh volcano brimmed with formidable furor.

While I sat nursing the baby in our glider, my mother-in-law set before me a neat array of breaded fish and sliced tomatoes, along with a fork. Seeing a sharp object near my child, my face crawled with hot tingles. I recoiled, as if I had been drenched in frying-pan grease. What if the fork flew into Noah's soft head?

My mothering instincts were strong, but this seemed like more than a desire to protect him. Rising out of nowhere, it was unwanted, disturbing, and uncontrollable. This was an intrusive thought. It ushered in a cascade of unruly images that taunted me into thinking I was a terrible mother. Only an evil being could imagine such gruesome pictures.

Throughout the day, the thoughts hounded me. My life became a constant peering out upon a danger-riddled world. Noah could tumble into the trash chute down the hall from our apartment. If I walked with him in a stairwell, I might slip and lose hold of him. Before, I barely noticed how close the cars were to pedestrians on the streets of Chicago. Now I pictured them skidding onto the sidewalk, and careening into my baby and me.

Indeed, our research indicated that close to 100 percent of people have the unwanted thoughts.

Dr. Jonathan S. Abramowitz,
a clinical psychologist and
international expert on OCD
and anxiety disorders

Locked in an endless what-if loop, I believed I was destined to be a prisoner of my irrational mind. The torment spun me into sobbing spells. I worried the thoughts would crowd out any remnants of sanity, and I might eventually lose my mind and hurt my child. But my tears soon gave way to frustration. I wanted a way out. "I have a lot of fight in me," I told my aunt visiting from Ohio. "I'm not giving up." Calling my OB/GYN was the first step I took to fend off the unwanted thoughts and confront the symptoms of postpartum obsessive-compulsive disorder (PPOCD).

Understanding Postpartum OCD

Prevalence, Symptoms, and Risk Factors

According to Dr. Jonathan S. Abramowitz,[16] a clinical psychologist and international expert on OCD and anxiety disorders, studies indicate that a higher-than-anticipated percentage of women with OCD say it starts—or their symptoms intensify—during pregnancy or the postpartum period: "In fact, among female OCD patients who have given birth, pregnancy and childbirth are the most commonly cited 'triggers' of OCD onset. Still, research suggests that postpartum OCD is fairly rare, probably affecting between 1% and 3% of childbearing women" (Abramowitz, n.d.).

Those numbers could be even higher, though. A *Journal of Reproductive Medicine* study (Miller et al., 2013) shows that 11 percent of the women it screened were positive for OCD symptoms at 2 weeks postpartum. At 6 months postpartum, almost half of the women had persistent symptoms, and an additional 5.4 percent had developed new OCD symptoms. The participants were more than 400 women who delivered children between June and September 2009 at Northwestern Memorial Hospital in Chicago. It is the first large study using a heterogeneous sample in a large metropolitan hospital to define the prevalence, clinical course, and risk factors for OCD symptoms in the postpartum period (Miller et al., 2013).

---

16 My personal communication with Dr. Jonathan S. Abramowitz took place between May 7, 2015, and July 16, 2015.

It's revelatory work.

Dr. Dana R. Gossett,[17] senior author of the study, says, "We found extremely high rates that I think are a little surprising." Gossett, chief of the division of obstetrics and gynecology at Northwestern University's Feinberg School of Medicine, points to the 11 percent figure as the highest number she has seen. She also says there is relatively little research on postpartum anxiety symptoms:

> It's only been in the last decade that anyone has paid any attention to peripartum psychiatric changes. Postpartum depression has had a number of champions, celebrities who choose to share their stories. So it has helped raise awareness and public pressure for research. I don't think OCD and anxiety have had that attention, and also they are less common. ... So postpartum anxiety and OCD are less publicly well-known, and also somewhat less prevalent. Combined, this makes them less of a priority.

Symptoms such as intrusive thoughts don't necessarily indicate the presence of a full-fledged disorder. Postpartum experts Karen Kleiman and Dr. Valerie Davis Raskin point out that a new mother only has a probable case of OCD if her worrying or obsessing inhibits her from functioning normally (2013).

Gossett experienced intrusive thoughts after her first child was born, about falling down the stairs or the baby rolling out of bed—but she didn't have postpartum OCD. "As a health care professional I recognized them as intrusive thoughts, which was not reassuring. It was quite disturbing," she says. "I think it's useful for women to know they're really common."

---

17   My personal communication with Dr. Dana R. Gossett took place between August 13, 2013, and April 11, 2016.

Among those who may be at higher risk of experiencing these thoughts are women who have a history of OCD, tend to be worriers, or describe themselves as overly analytical or perfectionistic. Those with no history of anxiety can also encounter them (The Postpartum Stress Center, 2010).

Obsessions and **compulsions** are the two dominant symptoms of PPOCD. **Obsessions**, also called **intrusive thoughts,** are persistent, repetitive thoughts or mental images usually related to harm coming to the baby, either accidentally or intentionally. Not having experienced them before, new mothers find them jarring and horrific. They realize their thoughts are irrational, and they're very unlikely to act on them (Postpartum Support International, n.d.).

Compulsions take place when a mother repeats actions to reduce fears and obsessions. Compulsive behavior might include cleaning, checking, counting, or reordering (Postpartum Support International, n.d.). New parents with OCD have reported mental compulsions, like praying over and over, and reassurance-seeking behaviors, such as researching symptoms online and asking others if bad thoughts about the baby are "normal" (Abramowitz, n.d.). Other compulsions include suppressing thoughts, or avoiding situations like taking the stairs or bathing the child (Miller et al., 2013). Some new mothers may also be hypervigilant when it comes to protecting the child (Postpartum Support International, n.d.).

OCD is an illness that can also take place outside the perinatal period (going forward, I refer to this as general OCD). General OCD differs from postpartum OCD in several ways:

▸ With general OCD, the onset is usually gradual and typically arises in late adolescence or early adulthood (Abramowitz et al., 2009). By contrast, postpartum OCD tends to surface quickly, sometimes within a week of childbirth (Abramowitz, n.d.).

▶ The nature of the obsessions and compulsions involved with general OCD are different, too, and commonly fall into five categories:

1. Obsessions about being responsible for causing or failing to prevent harm, checking compulsions, and reassurance-seeking;

2. Symmetry obsessions, and ordering and counting rituals;

3. Contamination obsessions, and washing and cleaning rituals;

4. Repugnant obsessions concerning sex, violence, and religion; and/or

5. Hoarding, which are obsessions about acquiring and retaining objects, and associated collecting compulsions (Abramowitz et al., 2009).

How Could I Think Such a Thing?

Intrusive thoughts related to the baby can be an indication of postpartum OCD. But even parents who don't have the disorder experience them. According to Abramowitz, nearly every new parent—mothers and fathers alike—gets intrusive thoughts. He headed a study that found 91 percent of mothers and 88 percent of fathers reported "distressing intrusive thoughts" about their babies at some point since the children were born (2006, p. 1368).

After the birth of his oldest daughter, Abramowitz was up late feeding the baby and thought to himself, "Nothing is stopping me from hauling off and hitting the baby." Abramowitz had never suffered from OCD, so it occurred to him that at some point, maybe every new parent experiences intrusive thoughts. He decided to conduct a study to find out. "Indeed, our research indicated that close to 100 percent of people have the unwanted thoughts," Abramowitz says—but because they're so difficult to discuss, not everyone reports them.

The thoughts run the gamut, from barely noticeable to unbearable, intermittent to constant, in the most severe cases pestering people by day or keeping them awake at night (J. S. Abramowitz, personal communication, July 16, 2015; The Postpartum Stress Center, 2010). Compulsive behaviors like constant checking or washing may or may not accompany the thoughts. Some examples of the thoughts are:

- ▸ "What if I drop my baby when I go down the steps?"
- ▸ "What if I slip and one of the knives falls on my baby?"
- ▸ "I think my family would be better off without me."
- ▸ "What if I put the baby in the oven?"
- ▸ "What if I drowned the baby?" (J. S. Abramowitz, personal communication, July 16, 2015; The Postpartum Stress Center, 2010).

The thoughts may also gnaw at a parent's self-worth, heaping on guilt and shame. They're powerful enough to make women feel as if they are bad mothers, crazy, or both. Kleiman refers to them as "scary thoughts." She founded The Postpartum Stress Center in Pennsylvania, a treatment and professional training center for prenatal and postpartum depression and anxiety. Kleiman reassures sufferers that they're not crazy, nor are they alone in their plight. According to The Postpartum Stress Center's website,

> If you are worried about the thoughts you are having, that's a good sign. Of course you're worried. It's a terrible burden to feel so attached and loving toward your baby and have such scary thoughts at the same time. Having these thoughts probably make [sic] you feel enormously guilty. ... But good mothers DO think bad thoughts when they are struggling with depression and anxiety (2010).

The center encourages mothers to do what's necessary to feel better. That might mean helping themselves with diversions, such as puzzles or other concentration games. Getting out of the house, dancing, and walking can serve as distractions. Sharing the thoughts with a trustworthy person can bring relief, as well (The Postpartum Stress Center, 2010).

OCD is NOT Psychosis

Postpartum OCD or symptoms of it are sometimes confused with postpartum psychosis. Both involve odd, violent thoughts, Abramowitz says, but that's where the similarities stop. Women with OCD are terrified of hurting their infants, and resist the thoughts by trying to dismiss them or neutralize them with another thought or behavior. The risk of someone with postpartum OCD harming her child is close to zero, he says (Abramowitz, n.d.).

A woman with psychosis, on the other hand, may see the thoughts—generally part of delusions—as consistent with her worldview, so she doesn't resist them. Thoughts of harming the baby may appear as a good idea.

> Postpartum psychosis is extremely rare, but because people with psychotic disorders sometimes act in accord with their delusions, postpartum psychosis poses very serious risks and often requires hospitalization to ensure the safety of the mother [and] infant (Abramowitz, n.d.; J. S. Abramowitz, personal communication, July 16, 2015).

Put another way, psychosis is a break with reality, says therapist and PMAD expert Diana Barnes. A woman may experience false beliefs about what's going on around her, and may hear critical and commanding voices, explains Barnes, who's also a past president of Postpartum Support International. "Sometimes the voices direct a mother to harm her child," she says.

Confusing postpartum OCD and psychosis and then misdiagnosing a patient can be harmful. Dr. Christina Hibbert, an Arizona-based clinical psychologist and expert on maternal mental health, writes,

> I have witnessed the unfortunate hospitalization of several mothers experiencing postpartum OCD. Misdiagnosed with Postpartum Psychosis, these mothers were seen as a threat to their infants and subsequently hospitalized in behavioral health units, placed on antipsychotic medication, and separated from their infants—many for up to a month or more. Most were also told they must stop breastfeeding, and some were reported to Child Protective Services (2014).

Once the women were released and they investigated their own symptoms, they located Hibbert or another expert in perinatal mental health. Only then did they receive the right diagnosis and treatment, including a referral for the proper medication and psychotherapy (Hibbert, 2014). A mother with postpartum OCD may delay treatment because she fears this very scenario: She will be diagnosed as psychotic, and her child will be taken away from her.

Before Abramowitz and his wife had their first child, they took a childbirth class where the instructor touched on postpartum mental health. When she explained that thoughts of harming the baby were always an indication of psychosis, Abramowitz approached her. "I was questioning a Mayo Clinic childbirth coach. But the truth is that I showed her the data, and [she] got it wrong," he says. He believes this type of misinformed instruction still occurs. In fact, some doctors don't understand the distinction. While postpartum OCD symptoms are very common, psychosis is a very rare condition.

Jennifer's Story

Intrusive thoughts can worm their way into some parents' worlds *before* a baby arrives. Jennifer Silliman[18] first experienced them in 2009, at the start of her third trimester of pregnancy with her daughter, Allyson. "My intrusive thought was an image of a very long, sharp knife stabbing my pregnant stomach," says Jennifer, an advocate and filmmaker. This was the only thought she had while pregnant, but it was corrosive. "I became obsessed about why I was having the thought. It was happening every minute, so I never had the thought out of my head during my third trimester." She researched her symptoms online and quickly self-diagnosed the thoughts as symptoms of OCD, but her doctors and nurses never mentioned the possibility of intrusive thoughts. Hoping the thoughts would vanish once the baby was born, she didn't share them with anyone.

Jennifer's pregnancy was high-risk because of placenta previa, a condition where the placenta hovers low in the uterus, partly or fully blocking the cervix. It can involve severe bleeding and threaten the lives of the mother and child, so doctors often schedule a C-section (National Library of Medicine, 2014). Jennifer's C-section was scheduled for mid-November. In early October, she began bleeding—the result of an extra lobe on her placenta—and was rushed in an ambulance to the hospital. There, she delivered Allyson, who aspirated when she was born and landed in the NICU.

As trying as her childbirth might have seemed, it was a welcome distraction: "The trauma gave me a break from the intrusive thoughts." She remained calm throughout the delivery and recovery, and wasn't jarred until she went to visit the baby in the NICU. Being near Allyson made her anxious. When the hospital released her after 5 days and without the baby, Jennifer

---

18 My personal communication with Jennifer Silliman took place between September 3, 2015, and September 17, 2015.

was relieved. Bringing the baby home terrified her. Still, she believed others would expect her to be upset by the prospect of going home without her child, so she played the part. Those around her offered encouraging words about the baby and how healthy she was: "If they only knew what was going through my head. No one was asking me about the intrusive thoughts."

Once home, the deafening din of intrusive thoughts continued, manifesting as images of knives stabbing the baby while she slept. Rather than voice the thoughts, Jennifer told her husband that she was plagued by postpartum depression. Because "postpartum depression" is a common-enough term, she believed it would suffice as an explanation, and she wouldn't need to relate her specific symptoms. She saw a therapist, a man with no training in perinatal mood and anxiety disorders, once or twice a week. They discussed everything but her intrusive thoughts: He didn't ask, and she didn't share.

The thoughts robbed Jennifer of regular enjoyment of her life. She avoided knives at almost all costs. She wouldn't use them to cut anything in the kitchen, and prepared a lot of soup instead of solid foods. When Christmas rolled around, she would tear gift-wrapping paper instead of cutting it with scissors. Soon, her thoughts turned suicidal, though she never made an attempt on her life.

Her breaking point surfaced when Allyson, a happy baby who slept and ate well, was 3 months old. Staring in the bathroom mirror one day, she thought, "I have no idea who this person is. I'm not enjoying motherhood." In a fearful torrent of tears, she fell to the floor.

> I finally told my husband everything that was going on. And pleaded with him not to take the baby, and not to leave me. The first thing he asked was if I wanted him to take all the sharp objects out of the house. He knew I wouldn't hurt anyone.

Jennifer called her therapist, who set up an emergency meeting for her with a psychiatrist in his practice. The psychiatrist diagnosed her with postpartum depression and postpartum OCD, and prescribed Luvox, medication used to treat OCD, and a very-low dose of Risperdal, an antipsychotic medication. Jennifer's mother has bipolar disorder, so she worried that she was experiencing it as well. But the psychiatrist reassured her that wasn't the case, and explained to her what the medication would do, and what the side effects might be. Within 3 days, the intrusive thoughts began to subside. She credits the psychiatrist with saving her life. "If I hadn't found that psychiatrist, who knows what would've happened? I was very lucky I found the right medicine the first time, and the right dose," she says. She stopped the medication after 2 ½ years, and hasn't gone back on it. "I don't have intrusive thoughts anymore. But my body is very sensitive to [violent] news stories, and things like that. So I'm more mindful of my body having gone through all of this."

Jennifer now works as a maternal mental health advocate. She created Moms-to-Moms, an online PMAD support group for mothers and fathers, and facilitates parenting classes for Healthy Mothers, Healthy Babies in Palm Beach County, Florida. The classes are geared to populations with high infant mortality rates. She also was the producer of the first American documentary to focus solely on maternal mental health, *Dark Side of the Full Moon*.

Treating OCD

According to Kleiman and Raskin,

> Postpartum OCD is probably the most underde-
> tected and undertreated of the anxiety disorders
> that follow childbirth, in part because women are
> embarrassed and reluctant to reveal what they
> are thinking. Women are often afraid to disclose
> the specific nature of their thoughts, because they
> fear being judged, misunderstood, labeled "crazy,"
> or—perhaps their greatest fear of all—they worry
> that their baby will be taken away (2013, p. 20).

OCD symptoms, particularly intrusive thoughts, are the disorder,
not the person, talking, according to Barnes. Too often, we fail to
distinguish between the illness and the person—something she
strives to reverse with her patients. Barnes says,

> I've had women say to me, "I'm a bipolar." But I say,
> "No, you're a woman who has bipolar disorder." ...
> If you have the flu and you've got a cough, you're
> identifying that as part of an illness. You're iden-
> tifying it as a symptom, not as something wrong
> with you. It's the same thing with psychiatric
> illness. But we're still in the Dark Ages about this.

Postpartum OCD responds to medications, particularly serotonin
reuptake inhibitors (SRIs), and cognitive-behavioral therapy (CBT)
(Abramowitz, n.d.; J. S. Abramowitz, personal communication,
June 25, 2015). Research indicates that these medications work
well for OCD:

- Luvox
- Zoloft
- Celexa
- Lexapro
- Prozac
- Paxil
- Anafranil
- Effexor (Jenike, n.d.).

CBT has proven more effective than medication for non-postpartum OCD, "so there's no reason to think that would be any different for postpartum OCD," Abramowitz says.

OCD is a mind-bending cycle, Abramowitz explains, where a person experiences an intrusive thought, misinterprets it as more meaningful than it really is, develops anxiety, and practices a compulsive behavior or ritual to quell the anxiety. But the compulsive behavior only ends up causing the intrusive thoughts to become worse and seem more meaningful. CBT strives to dismantle that cycle for the postpartum patient, using a four-step process:

1. **Assessment:** The therapist learns about the patient's obsessive thoughts, what triggers them, how they're interpreted, and how the person responds—for example, with compulsive behaviors.

2. **Education:** The therapist teaches the patient that almost everyone has intrusive thoughts around the time a baby is born. Problems arise when the person misinterprets the thoughts, which stirs anxiety.

3. **Cognitive therapy:** The therapist works with the patient to identify and challenge specific misinterpretations of intrusive thoughts. The therapist helps the patient consider evidence for and against her/his ideas that violent thoughts will lead to violent actions against her/his will.

4. **Exposure and response prevention (ERP):** The therapist helps a patient confront thoughts and situations that lead to anxiety and refrain from compulsive behavior. A mother afraid of bathing her newborn would practice doing so and realize that she's unlikely to hurt the baby (Abramowitz, n.d.).

Compulsive behaviors, as when a woman locks up all of her knives, or asks someone to watch as she bathes her child, are short-term fixes, Abramowitz says. People trick themselves into thinking they have to perform the rituals to avoid negative consequences, so it becomes a superstitious pattern. "In the long run, those rituals prevent the person from learning these thoughts are not a big deal," he says. CBT is a longer-term fix that leads patients to healthier thinking by showing them that whatever they've been afraid of is unlikely to happen.

The "active ingredient," Abramowitz says, is the exposure step: "You allow yourself to go there and say, 'It's okay.'" It also tends to be the most challenging part, because patients are afraid to confront their thoughts. He explains that,

> People with PPOCD conceal their thoughts. It becomes a dirty little secret and the person thinks, "It must be so awful and dark and deep." It just festers and gets worse and worse, whereas if you talk about it and let yourself go there, it normalizes these experiences. It helps the person develop a healthier relationship with their unwanted thoughts.

"CBT Changed the Way I Thought"

Cognitive-behavioral therapy helped Katie Kmiecik—who happens to be a therapist—rewire her relationship with her unwanted thoughts. After her daughter was born in March 2011, she experienced several perinatal mood and anxiety disorders, including PPD, PPA, postpartum OCD, and postpartum PTSD. As soon as the baby was born via C-section, she felt disconnected from her child. The baby spent a week in the neonatal intensive care unit (NICU), which intensified Katie's symptoms of the different PMADs.

Once home, Katie's symptoms of postpartum OCD raged, and centered on specific intrusive images:

▶ She worried that the baby would die, and she would think about planning the funeral, arranging the music, and emailing her coworkers with the news.

▶ She thought she would sexually abuse her baby, so she didn't want to change her diapers, bathe her, or dress her.

▶ She thought her husband would get killed in a car accident.

▶ She thought it was just a matter of time before a rapist or murderer would break into her house. So she made plans for how to deal with an intruder.

Katie developed compulsive behaviors around the intrusive thoughts, constantly checking the baby to make sure she was breathing, and that her face wasn't blue, as it had been three times while they were in the hospital. If her husband, mother, or sister were with her at home, she would ask one of them to bathe the baby or get her dressed. "I would think of myself as a sexual predator. I felt so ashamed and embarrassed. It took me a long time before I shared that with someone, because it was so embarrassing," she says.

Her sleep was compromised by dreams of the baby dying: "I had nightmares that she was in bed with us suffocating. I would wake up and frantically search for her in our bed until I realized she was in her crib."

After 6 months of suffering, she shared her agony with a close friend, and sought professional help the same day. She saw two therapists and one psychiatrist—all in different practices—and she was prescribed Zoloft and Wellbutrin for the depression and anxiety. One therapist used cognitive-behavioral therapy to treat her postpartum anxiety and OCD. The other addressed her postpartum PTSD with EMDR therapy. (For more on EMDR and Katie's PTSD story, see Chapter 2.)

Katie wasted no time launching into CBT. She worked dili-gently through all four steps, so she could get better as soon as possible. She attended therapy sessions twice a week, and did independent work at home, including reading. "CBT changed the way I thought," Katie says, and goes on to explain:

> In the cognitive therapy, some of my biggest anxi-eties were calmed as we looked at the evidence or lack thereof, for my catastrophic thoughts and for the scary thoughts I had about the baby. I then was given homework to practice on my own, counter-ing and replacing my negative thoughts with more realistic versions. This was the hardest step for me, because I didn't believe my positive replacement thoughts completely yet, but I trusted my therapist. This step changed me for the better to this day. I now practice replacing negative thoughts all the time about all different kinds of things! I'm much more relaxed and have less anxiety than I did even before my PMAD.

Her experience led her to focus her work as a therapist on mater-nal mental health. In 2013, she and her partners launched the Postpartum Wellness Center in Hoffman Estates, Illinois, which specializes in helping women and families affected by perinatal mood and anxiety disorders.

Speak Up

Intrusive thoughts are fiends we'd sooner flee than face down. But it's in confronting them that we diminish their power. One of the best ways of doing this is to talk about them. Jennifer Silliman attests to this. After being diagnosed with postpartum OCD by her psychiatrist, she continued seeing her therapist. She says,

> But he had a really hard time treating me for this [OCD] and knowing what to say. It almost made him equally uncomfortable to talk about it. He was very serious in telling me, "You better be careful who you share your story with."

He referred her to a support group. Finding nothing geared to maternal mental health in her area, she started a group of her own, Moms-to-Moms. At one of the first meetings Jennifer shared her intrusive thoughts, and noticed a woman who was upset. Afterward, the woman approached her and shared a similar experience. Her doctor had prescribed medication for intrusive thoughts, but she was afraid to fill it. Hearing Jennifer's story gave her courage to finally fill the prescription and start on a path to healing.

"If I can save someone's life by telling my story, then I will tell anybody and everybody my story, because they need to hear it," she says. Contrary to her therapist's advice, she saw that speaking up makes all the difference.

My intrusive thoughts centered on Noah. Like silent, macabre films on fast forward, they sent pulses of fear and dread zipping along my spine. Fortunately, they didn't interfere with my ability to take care of him. After a few days, I knew the thoughts weren't going away. One obsession focused on a frying pan hitting the baby's head. In my mind, it rang out this way: "What if the pan falls and hits Noah on the head? What if I hit him with it? Would I ever do that? Does this mean I'll hurt him? Am I crazy?"

I shared each thought with my husband. When I explained the frying-pan image, he laughed. I wasn't expecting him to laugh, but before long I was laughing too. The exchange proved cathartic, and allowed me to make light of the darkness creasing my brain.

Soon, I told my close family and friends. I wept one night, as I revealed the thoughts to my cousin.

"What should I do when I have those thoughts?" I asked.

"Nothing will happen," she said in a firm-but-loving tone. "You'll tell Matt, or you'll call me."

Not long after that conversation, I called my OB/GYN. I explained to her that I couldn't stop crying, and that scary, uninvited thoughts nagged me: "I feel like someone else has invaded my body and mind." She took me seriously and acted fast, suggesting talk therapy and antidepressants. "Your serotonin levels are probably low. The medication will boost them," my OB said. She prescribed sertraline, the generic form of Zoloft, and I picked it up from my pharmacy the same night.

She chose sertraline because it is believed to be safe to take while nursing, and because it treats symptoms of depression, OCD, and post-traumatic stress, which I was experiencing (Lanza di Scalea & Wisner, 2009; National Library of Medicine, 2014). It was important to start the medicine as soon as possible, not because she thought I was a danger to myself or to the baby. She wanted my quality of life to improve. Here was her keen bedside manner, as she tried to help me squeeze enjoyment from these otherwise arduous first days of motherhood.

After a short time of careful deliberation, I agreed to my OB's advised line of treatment. Within 10 days of starting the sertraline, the intrusive thoughts grew less frequent. My therapist, Rachel, was a licensed clinical social worker (LCSW) who allowed me to voice my thoughts and the anguish they bred. She wasn't alarmed, and assured me that many other women had tread similar paths.

Rachel didn't confuse the intrusions with psychosis, nor did she threaten to take my child or ring the authorities. The safer I felt, the more I talked.

My intrusive thoughts were silent scenes playing only for the eyes of my mind. Sharing them was like watching a film with others. We hit pause, replayed the scenes, and analyzed them, which underscored their absurdity and weakened their sway.

> *If I can save someone's life by telling my story, then I will tell anybody and everybody my story, because they need to hear it.*
>
> Jennifer Silliman,
> a mother, advocate, and
> filmmaker who battled PPD
> and postpartum OCD

I still experience intrusive thoughts, but they're less frequent. Because I know stress stirs them, one of my coping mechanisms is to manage the stress. That means regular exercise, eating clean foods, and getting at least 7 or 8 hours of sleep each night. Taking care of my body goes a long way to keeping my mind in shape.

Healing has come, bit by gradual bit. Sometimes, it surprises me. One such time was when my daughter, Syma, was born. My second time around the childbirth-bend, I was blessed with a near-flawless delivery. In the aftermath, I faced nothing more than a mild few days of the blues. No crying spells. No intrusive images. No postpartum *anything*. Syma's birth shifted my thinking in several ways:

▸ It showed me that I hadn't failed during Noah's birth, and propelled the process of me forgiving myself.

▸ It melted much of the sadness I still harbored from Noah's birth.

▸ It convinced me that new motherhood and joy aren't mutually exclusive.

Her arrival was a golden pillar in the fortress of my healing. It still shines in my memory as a source of hope and encouragement. My work on this book has also been a channel of healing. I now realize how common intrusive images are, not just for the postpartum woman, but for all new parents. Shared experience is a remarkable balm.

Considering the Causes

When it comes to explaining what causes postpartum OCD, experts discuss both biological and psychological considerations. On the biological side, research points to hormonal shifts as a potential culprit. For instance:

> Both estrogen and progesterone have been shown to affect serotonin pathways, and these hormones both exhibit dramatic falls in the immediate postpartum period. Other researchers have found that oxytocin, which is elevated in late pregnancy and in the postpartum period, is related to OCD symptoms (Miller et al., 2013, p. 119).

Serotonin is a neurotransmitter—a chemical naturally produced in the body that conveys nerve impulses across the gaps between nerve cells (Frey, 2012). When a person's brain produces serotonin, it reduces tension, and he or she feels less stressed, more focused, and relaxed (Darity, 2008). Abramowitz, however, raises several issues with the biological explanation:

> One difficulty I have with this model is that it doesn't explain why the obsessions in postpartum OCD tend to revolve around harm coming to the newborn baby, as opposed to concerning contamination, order, religion, or other common symptom themes in OCD. The environment must have an influence somewhere. It also does not explain why

almost all new mothers have unwanted infant-related thoughts, but only some develop clinical levels of OCD. But my most serious criticism of the biological approach to postpartum OCD is that it cannot explain that postpartum OCD can also occur in new fathers (who obviously do not experience the same hormonal fluctuation as do childbearing women) (Abramowitz, n.d.; J. S. Abramowitz, personal communication, July 16, 2015).

Along with Dr. Nichole Fairbrother, Abramowitz designed a psychological model of postpartum OCD. This model considers intrusive thoughts about a newborn to be a normal, harmless part of early parenthood. Problems arise only if a parent misinterprets the thoughts to mean that she or he will hurt the child. As to why someone might misinterpret intrusive thoughts as significant, Abramowitz says, "We think it has to do with the rapid increase in responsibility—which certainly is the case when one becomes a parent and gains the responsibility of caring for a helpless infant" (n.d.). Abramowitz continues his research at the University of North Carolina to better understand this question.

People with OCD also have difficulty with everyday levels of uncertainty that most people take for granted, according to Abramowitz. Feeling they have to know for sure, they strive for certainty—washing their hands, checking on the baby—and spend a lot of time doing it. "But that prevents them from learning to tolerate uncertainty in the long run," he says. This might stem from a learning history in which they were taught that anxiety or negative thoughts are bad.

The Power of Sharing

The Western world romanticizes new parenthood as a time of unparalleled charm and joy. In advertisements, glowing new mothers float, boasting flawless babies. Classes for first-time parents glaze over gritty realities. Many of us journey into this new phase of life equipped with little training in childcare. We tend not to realize how important it is to take care of ourselves, or how to recognize signs that we need help.

Having a child is a lot like throwing everything you own up in the air. When it falls down, you stare at the new shape of things with disbelief, wondering what to do. It ushers in one big era of unpredictability. Changes distort every aspect of our lives: relationships, eating, sleeping, going to the bathroom, finances, travel plans, grocery shopping, personal time, identity, self-worth. Not until this little person materializes does it become clear that he's real, and for the next however-many years, he's our responsibility.

Our brains swell. We might feel as if we're drowning as we try to absorb the watershed of life-in-flux. A different kind of normalcy takes a while to achieve, and it can be overwhelming and scary, but rarely is this mentioned. Such dialogue is beyond our culture's comfort zone. We afford little or no room for life's messes, like adjustment to motherhood, ubiquitous though they may be. So it shouldn't be surprising when women are blindsided by something like postpartum OCD. I'm not aware of any commercials featuring first-time parents who struggle in any way, let alone those who entertain unwanted thoughts of their children's demise.

To reverse this, we must share our stories. Words have the power to ease the poundings we take from intrusive thoughts. A woman who enters motherhood knowing these thoughts are universal might not be as alarmed as someone caught off guard. She should still pursue treatment if she believes it's necessary. But at least she does so feeling like a soldier backed by an endless throng of fellow fighters.

CHAPTER 5

Postpartum Psychosis

A Break With Reality

"Hope" is the thing with feathers –
That perches in the soul –
And sings the tune without the words –
And never stops – at all –

EMILY DICKINSON,
The Complete Poems of
Emily Dickinson, #254

While writing this book, I questioned how to cover post-partum psychosis. It is an intimidating subject—and a critically important one. The cases we often hear about involve a mother ending her child's life and/or her own. The theme of this book, though, is triumph and hope, not tragedy. Much of what we read and watch in the mainstream media emphasizes the cata-strophic side of mental illness in general, especially psychosis. It feeds the wild tide of sensationalism and fails to remind us of the many cases without a trace of tragedy, where women get proper treatment, heal, and go on to lead productive lives. The more I considered this, the more I believed I could help dispel the media-driven misperceptions that cloud our understanding of the illness.

Interviews with three women afflicted by postpartum psycho-sis—Sharon Gerdes, Teresa Twomey, and Melissa Bangs[16]—affirmed my belief. By retelling their stories, I could cover the illness and still convey hope. It's important to be aware of heart-breaking cases like the one involving Andrea Yates (Newman, 2006). They underscore the need to be educated on psychosis and swift in getting help. But they are not the norm. Focusing on them too intently can make us feel as if we're warring against an untamable foe. Far more stories of psychosis end well. They deserve just as much attention, and promise to shed new light on a misunderstood malady. As Teresa explains in her book, *Understanding Postpartum Psychosis: A Temporary Madness*, "[T]he vast majority of women who suffer this illness recover without hurting anyone, but they are largely in hiding—both historically and in present-day society" (Twomey, 2009, introduction, p. xxii).

This chapter reveals several such stories.

While postpartum psychosis is relatively rare, it is a severe illness. It's also temporary and treatable. Ideally, most women would be aware of their level of risk ahead of time. With timely,

---

16 See Chapter 8 for Melissa's story.

effective treatment, those suffering can go on to strong recoveries and full healing.

Teresa's Story

After her first child was born in 1998, Teresa Twomey[17] experienced postpartum psychosis and severe postpartum depression. At the time, she knew something was desperately wrong. But it wasn't until she was pregnant a second time that she realized her afflictions were perinatal mood disorders.

Know your risks. Get treatment from someone who understands reproductive mental health. If you don't feel safe, go to the hospital.

Dr. Diana Barnes, psychotherapist and PMAD expert

Hindsight rendered it somewhat obvious to her that she would be vulnerable to them. Before children, she struggled with anger, irritability, negative self-thoughts, and obsessing over the negative or about past experiences. Still, these didn't strike her as symptoms of depression, and she didn't know of a family history of the illness. Teresa says in her book,

> I would also have bouts of frenetic energy and insomnia—sometimes going for several days without sleep. But I did not think I had a "problem." I largely channeled my energy and anger and, to a large extent, learned to use it productively (p. 69).

She enjoyed a strong marriage with a loving, supportive husband with whom she planned to have her first child. Before children, she was a litigation attorney, and later a professional mediator, enjoying great success in her work. When she got pregnant, she

---

17 My personal communication with Teresa Twomey took place between November 3, 2015, and January 29, 2016. Much of what we discussed is also covered in her book. My account of her story draws on both my personal communication with her, and on her book.

was happily expectant. She took birth classes and read extensively on fetal development. She had a good relationship with her parents, and she considered herself a strong person. Postpartum depression, she thought, was something that happened to "other women"—those with serious mental or situational problems—and she doubts she had even heard of postpartum psychosis (p. 70).

> I did not fit the picture I had of women who might end up with postpartum mood disorders—so I didn't pay much attention to that. And when I developed PPP and postpartum depression, I was taken completely by surprise (p. 70).

Teresa endured a traumatic childbirth. She suffered extensive bleeding and a 3rd-degree tear, and went into a violent shaking spell afterward, during which she couldn't talk or move her right hand. When her midwife stitched her tear, she felt each searing movement of the needle. Once home, mobility was a painful challenge, making her feel trapped, and dependent on her husband and mother-in-law, who was visiting. Within a few days, she was worse. After meeting with the director of the center where she had her daughter, Teresa took antibiotics to fight the infection she had developed. Soon, she was on the mend, focused on recovery and caring for the baby.

The day before her mother-in-law was to leave, Teresa had her first intrusive image: As she passed a flight of stairs, she imagined throwing the child down it. Horrified and embarrassed, she couldn't bring herself to share the thought with her mother-in-law—nor did she know that intrusive thoughts plague almost all new parents, and they can be a symptom of postpartum OCD (for more about OCD, see Chapter 4).

As the intrusive thoughts persisted, Teresa avoided taking the stairs with the baby. She also developed paranoia. Worried the baby would stop breathing while she slept and die from sudden infant death syndrome (SIDS), she would check her, sometimes waking her up and causing her to fuss. She believed her husband was out to get her. As she writes in her book:

> I thought he wanted to divorce me and take our child. Although we talked about getting help, I secretly thought he was probably sabotaging our efforts. This man, who I trust more than anyone in the world, I felt I could not trust (p. 75).

Teresa had been raped as a teenager, and the birth of her daughter triggered symptoms of PTSD related to the rape. For instance, she had nightmares so horrid she would wake, awash in "sheer terror." The dreams weren't flashbacks to the rape, but images of her husband chasing her and trying to rape her with a knife.

Auditory hallucinations posed another persistent problem. During these, she heard someone come into the house, set down a briefcase, and shuffle papers. She would call her husband at work, and ask him to come home and investigate the noises. Time after time, he found nothing. Teresa writes,

> He thought I was hearing squirrels on the roof and grew very annoyed that I kept calling him to come home. I grew upset that he did not respond as quickly and seemed annoyed at me for calling him (which of course fed my paranoia). He did not say to me that he thought I was hearing squirrels, and I did not tell him the details of what I was hearing. Had either of us known about auditory hallucinations, maybe we would have explored this odd, recurring problem more thoroughly (p. 75).

Eventually, Teresa grew fearful of being alone with her daughter. She left a desperate message on her parents' answering machine, asking her mother to come to her side. Teresa's father retrieved the message, but didn't convey the gravity of it to her mother, so she didn't come. Unaware of the miscommunication, she perceived her mother's refusal to come as the ultimate abandonment. This too spurred her paranoia.

To drown out the auditory hallucinations, she kept the TV on, though she still experienced them. She didn't disclose how she couldn't follow the logical progression of a TV show, or that she couldn't read. Letters would be readable for only a few words, and then they looked like hieroglyphs to her. No matter how hard she tried to make sense of them, she couldn't. "That was particularly scary because I had never heard of such a thing before," Teresa writes (p. 76).

She also heard people talking and whispering. Sometimes the voices came from rooms that were empty or didn't exist. While she knew no one was there, she also worried these nonexistent people were conspiring against her.

Teresa's low point was a solitary visual hallucination in which she believed she had harmed her daughter.[18] Though it's difficult to explain the difference between this episode and the intrusive images, Teresa says that the two are distinct. She had no doubts about the intrusive images. They were simply thoughts in her mind, not something that actually happened. The visual hallucination seemed as if it were an event that took place, not just a thought. "When I recount this story to others, I cry. It is still so emotional because I remember it the way you would remember something that was real, even though I know it was not," she writes (p. 78).

The visual hallucination was the shortest part of her postpartum upheaval. Afterward, she sank into a severe depression. Teresa told those close to her that she couldn't "do this," and that she felt

---

18   Chapter 5 of Teresa's book covers this in detail. If you're in the midst of a perinatal mood disorder, please wait to read her descriptions until you feel they won't serve as triggers.

like a "bad mother," which she thought was the way to seek help. She didn't, however, share the specifics of what she experienced.

> And early on, even my medical provider had completely ignored my literally crying and blubbering that I was "not able to cope." So who do you tell, other than your family and doctor?

By 2000, she was pregnant with twin girls. While doing some research online, she had an exchange with a nurse and described her hallucinations. The nurse told her she was describing postpartum psychosis. That, in turn, stirred fears of what her second postpartum journey would be like. So Teresa shared some of her story with her family, as a way of helping them watch out for a possible recurrence. She told them that if her behavior or words were strange, or if she appeared agitated, they should immediately get her to a doctor. "And then the strangest thing happened, the twins were born, and I was fine," she writes (p. 80). During her second time, she was physically and mentally well.

Once through the psychosis, Teresa encountered significant emotional turmoil over the fact that she had the illness, something she calls "post-recovery recovery." She writes, "I searched for reasons *why* this would happen to me. I grieved the lost quality time with my daughter. I had to learn to trust myself again" (p. 80).

She believes that if she had knowledgeable medical providers and caregivers, if they had done a thorough analysis of her history, and if she had been examined about her mood after childbirth, her situation would have been different. "It is absurd that it is not *routine* to evaluate postpartum women for mood disorders, particularly those who had experienced trauma or have complications," she writes (p. 81).

Teresa says her mental health is stronger than ever. She thrives on being a mother to three girls, and she's focused on serving as an advocate for perinatal mood disorders, particularly psychosis.

As part of her work, she strives to educate women and their families. The most important thing to remember is "It can happen to you or someone you love. It can happen to any woman, anyone you'd think of as an otherwise ordinary woman. It's not predictable." While there are risk factors that can suggest whether someone is more or less at risk, it's impossible to say a woman faces no risk.

She believes some facets of her character are stronger because she endured postpartum psychosis. Since she had a mild case, her story offers more positive than negative.

Understanding Postpartum Psychosis

Prevalence, Symptoms, and Risk Factors

Compared to postpartum depression or anxiety, postpartum psychosis is relatively rare. Out of every 1,000 deliveries, it strikes between one and two mothers, and the onset is generally within 2 weeks of birth (Postpartum Support International, n.d.). Symptoms can include:

- ▶ delusions or strange beliefs;
- ▶ hallucinations, which involve seeing and/or hearing things that aren't there;
- ▶ irritability;
- ▶ agitation/restlessness;
- ▶ inability to sleep or diminished need for it;
- ▶ paranoia and suspiciousness;
- ▶ rapid mood swings; and/or
- ▶ difficulty communicating at times (D. L. Barnes, personal communication, February 11, 2016; Postpartum Support International, n.d.).

Risk factors of most significance are a personal or family history of bipolar disorder, or a past psychotic episode. Among those who develop postpartum psychosis, the rate of suicide is about 5 percent, while the infanticide rate is around 4 percent. These tragedies arise because the women have a split with reality. Delusions and strange beliefs seem normal to them. They frequently have a religious overtone, but not always. It's vital for these women to get immediate medical care from professionals trained in treating postpartum psychosis (D. L. Barnes, personal communication, February 11, 2016; Postpartum Support International, n.d.).

Like Teresa Twomey, many women who survive psychosis don't have delusions that command them to behave violently. Delusions come in many forms, and not all are destructive. (See the side-bar in this chapter, "Delusions: A Primer.") Most survivors don't hurt themselves or anyone else. Yet, the threat exists. If a new mother exhibits any of the symptoms above, family and friends should quickly get her into the care of a perinatal mental health professional (D. L. Barnes, personal communication, February 11, 2016; Postpartum Support International, n.d.).

Dr. Diana Barnes, a psychotherapist who specializes in women's reproductive mental health, has consulted as an expert witness on cases of infanticide where postpartum psychosis has been at issue. She says a new mother must know her risks, and so should her partner, and those close to her. Any mental illness with psychotic symptoms places a woman at increased risk, according to Barnes. "It can be a family or a personal history of bipolar disorder, or of schizophrenia, which has psychotic symptoms, or of schizoaffective disorder, or major depressive disorder with psychotic features."

Routine screenings of women during pregnancy will uncover such risks (for more on screening, see chapters 6 and 9). "Although [postpartum] psychosis is a serious illness, it is a treatable illness. The problem arises when the illness is misdiagnosed and when it is overlooked. That's when we start to read these horrible stories in the newspaper," Barnes says.

If there is a takeaway message, she says, it's two-fold. Postpartum psychosis is neither to be ignored, nor is it to be feared: "Know your risks. Get treatment from someone who understands reproductive mental health. If you don't feel safe, go to the hospital."

Delusions: A Primer

Delusions are fixed beliefs in something that is not true. They can be either bizarre or non-bizarre. Bizarre delusions are implausible. They don't derive from ordinary life experiences, and others can't understand them. An example of a bizarre delusion is when a person believes that some external force has removed his or her internal organs and replaced them with someone else's organs without leaving wounds or scars. Non-bizarre delusions are plausible, but lacking evidence. Examples of non-bizarre delusions could be the beliefs that one is under surveillance by the police, or that a significant other is being unfaithful (American Psychiatric Association, 2013; Bressert, 2016; D. L. Barnes, personal communication, February 11, 2016).

The content of delusions can take on different themes:

- ▸ **Persecutory:** One will be harmed, harassed, etc., by an individual, organization, or other group
- ▸ **Referential:** Certain gestures, comments, environmental cues, etc., are directed at oneself

> ‣ **Grandiose:** Someone believes she or he has exceptional abilities, wealth, or fame
>
> ‣ **Erotomanic:** A person falsely believes that someone else is in love with her or him
>
> ‣ **Nihilistic:** A major catastrophe will happen
>
> ‣ **Somatic:** Someone with these is preoccupied by health and organ function (American Psychiatric Association, 2013).

Sharon's Story

Sharon Gerdes[19] developed postpartum psychosis after the birth of her second child in 1979. Back then, little was known about the illness and how to treat it, says Sharon, a former public relations chair and vice president of Postpartum Support International. The military hospital where she delivered her son was probably even less informed than mainstream hospitals.

Her husband, who then served in the U.S. Air Force, was out of the country when she went into labor. Her mother, who was working and had health issues, was unable to be with her. During labor, the nurses weren't attentive to Sharon's appeals for help. An example of this is when she borrowed a watch from someone to time her own contractions. Her son was born 6 weeks prematurely, and weighed just 3 ½ pounds. The stress of not knowing if the baby would live or die weighed heavily on her. She believes she

---

19   My personal communication with Sharon Gerdes took place between September 21, 2015, and February 26, 2016.

had some symptoms of postpartum PTSD, but she didn't know it at the time.

Because she wanted to nurse her son, she opted to stay in the hospital and pump milk for him. She pumped regularly. Nurses floated in and out to check her vital signs, and she had a roommate. None of this afforded her much time for rest. At night, she was unable to sleep. Sharon developed symptoms of psychosis, and detailed them in her personal journal. She was euphoric and out of touch with reality. She calls it a religious feeling that God had appointed her to do something important, and she believed irrational things—that she'd invented a new language, and that others could read her mind. Thoughts of harming herself or the baby never occurred to her.

She reached her limit after 11 days: "I really thought the doctors and nurses weren't taking good care of me or my son. I wanted to transfer to a different hospital." Angry, desperate, and determined to take the baby and leave, she shared this with a nurse, who refused her request. At that point, Sharon slapped the nurse. She was placed in a straightjacket and taken to the county mental ward, where she was placed under the care of a psychiatrist, who prescribed her antipsychotic medication. She refused medication, and it took five medical staffers to restrain and medicate her: "Two weeks later, I could barely talk or walk or control my bladder."

After those 2 weeks, she returned home, and took the medication for around two or three months. Though she no longer felt psychotic, she was "slightly out of touch with reality," until she re-established a normal pattern of sleep. Because of the time apart from her son, and a concern that the medication might transfer to him through her breast milk, Sharon was unable to resume nursing, which saddened her.

At one point, she had a mild relapse. Her psychiatrist suggested she start taking lithium, and he believed she would be on it for the rest of her life: "I rejected his diagnosis. I was fine and happy before the childbirth—normal. So I refused to take the medication." Sharon believes her psychosis was kicked up by a combination of factors: not knowing if her son would live or die when he was born so small, and a lack of sleep and social support. "If either my husband or mom had been there to support me emotionally, I wouldn't have had the psychosis." Social support from family, friends, and other mothers is critical to all new mothers, particularly those who face trauma in the sensitive time surrounding childbirth.

When it comes to assessing a woman's risk and determining the roots of her illness, Sharon says, mental-health professionals often overlook the impact of a traumatic experience. Whether it involves her own physical struggles, a life-threatening condition for her baby, or difficulty with nursing—if a mother perceives her situation as traumatic, it is. The trauma can affect her mental health and factor into psychosis. If you're dealing with trauma related to childbirth, ask for help. Tell someone you trust, such as a partner, friend, family member, doctor, nurse, or therapist. Let them know how the trauma has affected you.

As to her recovery, Sharon says, "It was 6 months of crawling my way back to sanity. It took me about three years to get over the incident and get on with my life." The psychosis contrasted starkly with her past successes: flourishing in her college career and later, as a certified food scientist. "It really took a long time for my psyche to heal." She currently runs an international consulting firm, working with major food corporations on product development, nutrition, and regulatory issues.

Sharon is stronger and more empathetic because of her journey through postpartum psychosis. While she was in the mental hospital, she had no money or freedom. When another patient with a can of soda passed it around the group, she took a sip—and felt humiliated because she couldn't buy her own: "When you're always a winner and you've never been on the bottom, you don't have much empathy for others who might be experiencing mental illness, or suicide, or other setbacks in life."

She wrote a novel, *Back in Six Weeks*, inspired by her experiences. When she started to write, she planned to publish it under a pen name. Just before publication in 2014, colleagues suggested she use her real name, to make the book more powerful and help reduce the stigma of postpartum psychosis. So she did.

Education and Treatment

Assessing women's risks for developing psychosis, educating them and their families on the illness, and providing proper treatment—these aren't just important steps to fight the illness. These efforts save lives.

Women and their partners must be familiar with the symptoms of psychosis and how it manifests, Barnes says. It's especially important for those closest to the new mother. They're in the best position to notice a difference in her behavior. If she's in a psychotic state, she won't necessarily identify it as such—it may seem to her like a reasonable reality. A woman with depression usually knows her thoughts are awry. A woman plagued by psychosis, however, might not have that insight. "You can't talk someone out of a delusion if they're in a psychotic state," Barnes says.

Teresa Twomey believes educating people about psychosis is the most important thing we can do:

> Not just for the woman, but for her family, because
> they are her first line of defense. And this can come
> on fast, so that's important. Unless everyone has
> a better understanding of this illness, we'll say,
> "Who would've thought?"

In her advocacy work, Teresa often fields calls from people seeking help for a loved one with postpartum psychosis. Instead of getting formal treatment, they just want to keep a close eye on her. They explain that she's not the type of person to hurt anyone. This assumption indicates a lack of knowledge about the illness. "It doesn't mean she's not at risk if she's a loving person."

Teresa cautions those who opt to care for a woman without professional help. "You have to have people awake with her 24/7 who can overpower her. Not in another room—with her, awake in the same room, if you're going to have her and the baby there," she says. If they can't maintain round-the-clock monitoring, she raises a question for them: "Can you live with the worst-case scenario?" Because most people aren't able to provide their loved one with constant care, she urges them to get professional help.

Many women Barnes has encountered don't have access to the level of care they need. Problems run the gamut, from women who seek care and are misdiagnosed, to women whose treatment is too brief. Then there are the barriers created by stigma. "There is so much emphasis on the awful things that happen when a woman has psychosis. It's so terrifying that it prevents some women from actually seeking out treatment," she says. They're afraid that if they share with others about voices they're hearing, they'll be perceived as crazy, and someone will take their children away.

Teresa attests to this. She writes in her book, "Too often women do not tell others what they are suffering. I didn't. Like many women, on one hand I feared that I would not be believed; on the other hand I feared the stigma of mental illness" (p. 82). So she hid it, and barely survived during her 2 years of pain.

Treatment

Although Sharon Gerdes learned a lot during her encounter with postpartum psychosis, her level of care wasn't optimal:

"My treatment was far from ideal, [in terms of] both the physical and emotional impact. It was devastating to me."

Sharon thinks she may have fared better if she had been treated with medication to restore her sleep patterns before receiving antipsychotic medication. This approach—treating patients first with sleep medication before administering other drugs—is suggested by a study published in 2015, on postpartum psychosis and mania. She says,

> I believe that if the first step in this protocol had been used, I might have had a much shorter treatment time and an overall much better outcome. Still, I was very fortunate as I realize the situation could have been much worse.

The study was conducted at the mother-baby unit of the Erasmus Medical Center in Rotterdam, the Netherlands. It says that because the illness is unpredictable and has severe symptoms, treatment with medication is typically immediate: "Unfortunately, however, few standardized treatment recommendations are currently available for postpartum psychosis, as research has been limited and no randomized trials have been conducted" (Bergink et al., 2015, p. 115).

Authors of the study treated and evaluated 64 women with postpartum psychosis or mania, both during their stay in the medical center and at the 9-month mark after their babies were born. Treatment consisted of medication as well as "nonpharmacological interventions to optimize mother-baby interaction," including feedback from nursing staff, baby massage, and video-interaction guidance (Bergink et al., 2015, p. 117). The medication was administered in a four-step process:

1. During the first 3 days, all patients were solely treated with sleep medication, benzodiazepines. The goal was to first address sleep loss—an important factor in postpartum psychosis—and determine if restored

sleep leads to clinical remission of manic and psychotic symptoms.

2. If manic or psychotic symptoms continued, antipsychotic medication was suggested starting on the fourth day, in combination with the sleep medication.

3. If there wasn't significant improvement after 2 weeks of treatment on the antipsychotic and sleep medication, lithium was added to the treatment mix.

4. For patients who didn't improve after 12 weeks on the combination of sleep medication, antipsychotic, and lithium, electroconvulsive therapy (ECT) was recommended. Before starting ECT, all psychotropic medications would be tapered to a halt (Bergink et al., 2015).

All but one of the 64 women achieved full clinical remission during the first three steps. The remaining patient was discharged against medical advice during step three, and didn't go into remission during the 9-month follow-up period. Symptoms for most of the women—47—remitted after step three; step two was sufficient treatment for 12 others, and the remaining four recovered after step one. At 9 months postpartum, 51 of the 64 women were still in remission.

The authors offer a variety of recommendations for treatment, in terms of general strategies, medication, and ECT. They make several important, if often overlooked, suggestions, including focusing on the woman's sleep patterns and her interaction with her baby, and providing support for the father. They also point out that treating a patient in a "mother-baby unit is associated with improved patient satisfaction and may help reduce time to recovery." (See Chapter 9 for more on mother-baby units.)

Sharon Gerdes believes women with postpartum psychosis don't always receive the best possible treatment, because their care providers incorrectly diagnose them, particularly with bipolar disorder. For some, it's the correct diagnosis—but not for everyone. A woman who experiences a traumatic childbirth, for example, and then weathers the typical postpartum storm of hormonal changes, sleep deprivation, and general life upheaval may find herself drowning in psychosis. Once she receives proper treatment and heals, she may no longer need medication. "Some women can make a complete recovery," Sharon says. "You can move beyond this and have a normal, healthy, happy life."

The Netherlands study echoes Sharon's sentiments:

> [S]ome patients may have a biological vulnerability to severe affective psychosis that is limited to the postpartum period. The postpartum period is well established as having a dramatically elevated risk for affective instability and psychosis; the risk during the postpartum period is estimated to be 20–25 times higher than during other periods. Moreover, several studies have demonstrated that over long follow-up periods, a sizable proportion of women show no evidence of mania or psychosis outside the postpartum period (Bergink et al., 2015, p. 121).

Too often women do not tell others what they are suffering. I didn't. Like many women, on one hand I feared that I would not be believed; on the other hand I feared the stigma of mental illness.

Teresa Twomey,
postpartum-psychosis survivor and
PMAD advocate

Setting the Record Straight

It is important that we do not blame postpartum psychosis—or any PMAD—for wrong behavior. An example of this cropped up as I wrote this chapter. I highlight this instance not to point fingers, but to show how a lack of understanding can mislead others, especially those with little or no exposure to mental illness.

A television reporter mentioned postpartum psychosis while covering the terror attacks that took place in San Bernardino, California (Whitlock, 2015). One of the two terrorists was a wife and mother of a 6-month-old child. During an on-air interview with two former FBI agents, Jim Clemente and Robert Chacon, the reporter inquired about the woman's motives. After Clemente explained that she had been radicalized, that she had trained and prepared for the attacks, the reporter continued, asking Clemente, "But I just have to ask you, could there be something else, anything else, that could have explained her involvement? Something like a postpartum psychosis?" Clemente replied, "Well, postpartum psychosis, in the cases that I've seen of it really is typically internal. I mean, the violence goes internally or within the family." He went on to say that children are most likely the ones harmed, or the person suffering the illness. "So, I don't see this as a common case of postpartum psychosis. This is something much more related to extremism" (Whitlock, 2015).

The reporter's question sent palpable shudders down the spine of the postpartum community. TV-based journalists wield the giant mouthpiece and bright lights of television news. They have the power to inform or misinform the masses. In this case, I believe viewers were misled when the reporter linked postpartum psychosis and terrorism. The connection is inaccurate and unfair. It casts women suffering from psychosis into deeper, darker shadows, and intensifies stigma's already caustic burn.

Postpartum psychosis is a serious mental illness. It can be deadly. It is also temporary and treatable, and many women overcome it. They are not terrorists. If you find yourself engaged in a conversation about psychosis, remember Sharon Gerdes, Teresa Twomey, and others like them. More and more women are sharing their stories of perinatal mental illness. They summon help, rebound in remarkable ways, and lend hope to others who struggle. Point to these stories, and to their triumphs and lessons. We can build on them to improve treatment and care, to expedite recovery and full healing.

The coverage I mentioned above affirms what we already know. The world needs more educated conversations on maternal mental health. We should have these talks until the truth becomes second nature. The world needs to hear the voices of women who have battled the illnesses. It needs to hear the voices of the clinicians and therapists, who treat them and work diligently on their behalf. It needs to hear the voices of the friends and family, who hold their hands, wipe their tears, and remind them they are worth far more than what they're feeling or thinking on any given postpartum day. This is how we will change things—one voice at a time, dispelling pesky myths that perpetuate. In time, our voices will build a chorus that resounds so powerfully, it can't be ignored.

CHAPTER 6

Shaking Off the Shame

How to Confront Stigma

You may not control all the events that happen to you, but you can decide not to be reduced by them.

MAYA ANGELOU,
Letter to My Daughter

Antidepressants, as they tinker with the delicate balance of the mind, spell uncertainty. Only people who are gravely ill or weak-willed need them. That's what I thought—until my OB/GYN prescribed one to help treat my PPD. The idea of mood-altering medication became even scarier to me then. I worried that it would seep into my breast milk, and affect Noah. I didn't believe it could stop the seemingly endless tide of tears and dark thoughts. My brain was permanently warped. It had to be. Matt was leery, too, and he asked me to seek his mother's opinion. I didn't want to though. What would she think? As a missionary in France, she had raised four children, but she hadn't faced a perinatal mood disorder. I assumed she would see it as a stain on my reputation. Maybe she would wonder if her son had married the wrong person.

Wishing I could call *my* mother, I steeped in self-pity for a day or so. I wanted counsel from someone familiar, someone who would love me despite my shortcomings. I called my dad. He was supportive, but he couldn't offer a mother's perspective.

Whether or not Matt's mother would think the worst of me, she had a wealth of experience that could help. She's quite kind, and I knew her advice would put Matt at ease. I had to do whatever it would take to protect my family, and that included sharing my symptoms with other trustworthy people.

So I called her.

She encouraged me to try the medication, and to consider it a step on the way toward wellness. I'm fortunate to have a loving, empathetic mother-in-law. Despite my depressed state, I didn't unfairly demonize her or convince myself that she would respond harshly. PMADs can distort otherwise clear thought patterns and make us more vulnerable, even to the stigma we inflict on ourselves.

I started the antidepressant, sertraline, and within 10 days, my crying spells vanished. The scary thoughts, which can be a symptom of postpartum OCD, grew less frequent (The Postpartum Stress Center, 2010). My therapist aptly suggested that the medication would stop me from feeling as if I were sinking into quicksand. That's just what it did. As I regained ground, I knew I wasn't crazy. I was fighting an illness, and I began to believe I would recover.

After I interviewed other women about their encounters with perinatal mood disorders, I considered my bout to be relatively short-lived. That was due to several factors:

▸ I acted fast on what was within my control—asking for help, seeing a therapist, trying an antidepressant;

▸ My body and mind responded well to the line of treatment I pursued; and

▸ God shared some of His grace with me.

Each woman's story is as distinctive as her fingerprints. She may have a mood disorder for a few months, a few years, or longer. What worked for me wouldn't necessarily work for someone else, even if she confronted similar situations or symptoms. A new mother shouldn't compare herself to anyone else. She should strive only to find the support that will lead to healing for *her* mind and body.

Why are we afraid of mental illness? Who knows. The stigma associated with mental illness is bad enough, but when you attach it to motherhood, it is combustible.

Karen R. Kleiman, postpartum-depression expert, author, and founder of *The Postpartum Stress Center in Pennsylvania*

Stigma Most Unkind

Like other illnesses, perinatal mood and anxiety disorders are temporary and treatable. PMADs are different because they plague the mind, not the body. "Mental illness" is a stigma-laden phrase. It terrifies many, including new mothers. Afraid of what others will think if they reveal their symptoms, they suffer in silence and don't seek help. We use the word "stigma" a lot. *Webster's New World College Dictionary* defines it as "something that detracts from the character or reputation of a person, group, etc.; mark of disgrace or reproach" (Neufeldt & Guralnik, 1997, p. 1316). By attaching stigma to mental illness, we insult those who suffer, branding them disgraceful.

Crystal Clancy,[20] a licensed marriage and family therapist (LMFT) who specializes in perinatal and reproductive mental health, developed postpartum depression and anxiety after the birth of her second child, a girl, in 2005. "I felt like a failure to both my older child and to my newborn. I felt like I had to hide how much I was struggling to everyone else because I am a therapist, and told myself I 'should' be able to handle things just fine," says Crystal, co-director of Pregnancy and Postpartum Support Minnesota. "On the surface, I was presenting myself as a competent, confident mom."

She didn't cry much or feel suicidal, but she was irritable, frustrated, and emotionally detached from the baby. Beyond meeting her daughter's basic needs, she didn't interact with her. "I would feed her, change her diaper, put her in her bouncy seat, and let her hang out a lot." She also had escapist fantasies:

> I did have a plan at one point to leave, to put my
> daughter down for a nap knowing my husband
> would be on his way home from work, take my

---

20 My personal communication with Crystal Clancy took place between November 1, 2012, and May 11, 2016.

> older child, and leave. We would go for 6 months,
> and stay somewhere and come back, and she would
> be older and things would be better. I didn't want
> to die, hurt myself, or her. I just wanted to leave.

She believes her depression lifted when the baby was about 6 or 7 months old, and gave way to anxiety. But Crystal didn't seek help until her daughter was nearly 2 years old. She went to her nurse-midwife, who prescribed the antidepressant Lexapro. Within 3 days, she started feeling better. She was less irritable and better able to enjoy her daily life. In retrospect, she wishes she had gotten help sooner.

Crystal has tried to stop taking Lexapro, but she continues using it because, "I did not like who I was off the medication. My kids and husband didn't like who I was." She also sleeps better and hasn't had side effects.

In addition to the medication, she believes a vital part of her healing came through her work as a therapist. It has given her a better understanding of her own postpartum battles, and allows her to use what she learned to help other women fight and beat PMADs.

Mothers hide their agony out of shame, hoping the symptoms will vanish, according to Karen Kleiman. Almost 20 years after the first publication of their book, *This Isn't What I Expected: Overcoming Postpartum Depression*, Kleiman and Dr. Valerie Davis Raskin reported that stigma remains strong:

> [W]omen with PPD continue to wait apprehensively in the dark corners of their lives, fearful of judgment, stigma, ridicule, and misdiagnosis. They wait, hoping this will go away by itself, hoping they will not go completely mad, hoping they do not have to let anyone know how they are really feeling (2013, introduction, p. x).

As a way of coping, a new mother becomes expert at looking and sounding fine, Kleiman says. So no one wonders if, for example, she might be suicidal.

> Why are we afraid of mental illness? Who knows. The stigma associated with mental illness is bad enough, but when you attach it to motherhood, it is combustible. It's supposed to be a great time. [Saying] "No, actually I feel like hell"—no one wants to hear that. So we suck it up and we pretend. The stigma is a big question, and no one has a good answer for it.

A Lack of Doctors in the Know

Talking with health care providers about perinatal mood disorders is a major hurdle for women. Some say they feel like they're in limbo after the baby is born. They no longer pay regular visits to their OBs, and pediatricians are focused on the child's health. Finding a doctor with whom they're willing to share their most vulnerable thoughts and feelings can be a daunting task.

Another challenge lies in educating doctors, so they know the right questions to ask new mothers. Dr. Christina Hibbert, who founded the Arizona Postpartum Wellness Coalition, a nonprofit that educates women, families, and providers on perinatal mental health, says it's difficult to get doctors to participate in trainings. She has conducted trainings across the state of Arizona since 2005, and continues to do at least one every year, for medical and mental-health providers including nurses, OB/GYNs, pediatricians, counselors, psychologists, psychiatrists, and home-workers.

Hibbert finds that doctors give excuses as to why they can't attend. Others register but don't show up. Nurses "are better about getting the education, but doctors are tough. The doctor may not have all the information a mom needs [on PMADs], but a nurse might," she says. Perhaps doctors believe they already know everything they need to know, so they don't pursue more education, according to Hibbert. Although OBs and pediatricians may talk more about PMADs now than in the past, it doesn't mean they know the specifics, such as distinguishing between postpartum OCD and psychosis. "I still have so much to learn, and I am a specialist in it," she says. "If we are not getting as much education as possible, we are doing patients a disservice."

Doctors often don't ask the right questions, and even when they do, women aren't comfortable revealing how they feel, Kleiman says:

> Mom is still afraid if she talks about how bad she feels, at best she will be misunderstood, and at worst someone will take away her baby. She might say she is not feeling good. But she may hide the extent to which her distress is interfering with her day.

It isn't easy, even for health care providers who ask the right questions and offer support. They hear a mother say she has scary thoughts, but unless they're specially trained in and educated about PMADs, they don't know what to do, according to Kleiman. A good rule of thumb, she says, is this: If a woman is complaining of symptoms and she is beyond 2 or 3 weeks postpartum, she does not have the baby blues.

The Best of Times, the Worst of Times

New motherhood is depicted as one of the best times in a woman's life, but only half of us find that it lives up to its image (Kleiman & Raskin, 2013). The radiant mothers advertised in popular media are an impossibly sunny act to follow. We shouldn't be surprised when a woman with postpartum depression thinks she isn't measuring up to such a standard. Afraid of what others will think if she appears to veer from society's norms, she hides her struggle. Instead of seeing a mood disorder for what it is—a sticky patch along the way—she believes it will define the *rest* of the way, and who she is.

Kleiman, who has worked with women and their families for nearly 30 years, says a new mother contends with a unique set of circumstances:

- There is a new human being in the picture—a baby—and she must protect and support that life.

- She is sleep-deprived.

- She must juggle the many demands of the transition to motherhood.

According to Kleiman:

> These feelings like, "I am overwhelmed. I should have not had the baby. I am powerless. I am totally out of control," those are expressed as symptoms to you and me, but they are experienced as self to her. When a woman says she has a sore throat or a fever, the doctor says, "Let's treat it accordingly." But when a woman has postpartum depression, she says, "I suck as a mother. I want to kill myself. I can't live one more day like this. I can't be who I am." When I hear a woman say that, I hear her like she is saying [she has] a sore throat.

For a while, I believed the symptoms of my mood disorder defined me. I worried that I wouldn't measure up to society's standards, and wondered what others would think when I told them I had unstoppable crying spells. But stigma—either from myself or others—didn't scare me into silence. I offered my story to anyone who would listen, and it brought me great relief. It was the first step I took on the road to healing.

Lucy,[21] a PPD survivor, was afraid of being labeled "crazy." A mother of two, she had postpartum depression after the birth of her first child, a boy, in 2005. For 6 months, she denied any trouble. Though she knew things weren't right, she didn't think she had a treatable illness, nor did she realize it was postpartum depression. "I thought maybe I just couldn't handle having a newborn. Or that I had 'baby blues' and sleep deprivation. So I guess you could say I thought it was an identity flaw," Lucy says.

She believes that postpartum depression is often treated as a red flag, especially by health care professionals, and that people with mental-health problems are punished: "Now, anytime I'm feeling off, the postpartum depression is a big crazy mark. And that was part of why I didn't want to get meds with my son, and why it took me so long to get meds." Lucy was on medication for 6 months, and then she was fine.

Before her son was born, she quit her job as a professional organizer. She didn't earn enough to justify hiring a nanny, and she was excited about becoming a mother, so the choice was easy. "I had always babysat/nannied. I really thought it was going to be easy. That I would be tired, but able to handle the task of caring for an infant." Like so many of us, she was taken by surprise. She says,

> Postpartum depression made me feel angry and resentful toward my husband. I also kept thinking, "I made my bed, now I have to lie in it." I did not feel any anger toward my baby. It was all directed either inward or at my husband.

---

21   Lucy's real name has been changed to protect her privacy.

She felt trapped, stuck at home with the baby while her husband went off to work. Meanwhile, breastfeeding was a major challenge. The baby didn't latch properly. She was caught in an endless loop of nursing, pumping, and tending her stage-three tear: "I feel like I never even saw the baby. And the baby was not a sleeper. To this day, a crying baby initially sends a chill up my spine and I think, 'He will never sleep again.'"

I felt like a failure to both my older child and to my newborn. I felt like I had to hide how much I was struggling to everyone else because I am a therapist, and told myself I 'should' be able to handle things just fine.

CRYSTAL CLANCY, co-director of Pregnancy and Postpartum Support Minnesota, who developed postpartum depression and anxiety after the birth of her second child

Nursing was severely painful, and her body didn't yield enough milk—but she was determined, and went through a number of hospital-grade pumps. Pumping "felt like a prison," she says, because of its repetitive nature—30 minutes at a time, several times a day: "I even got up to pump at night while my husband fed our son a bottle. It felt like drudgery, and I had no joy at all in caring for my son."

Lucy eventually stopped nursing. She didn't pursue it with her second child, something she doesn't regret. "I was still tired all the time, but I had so much fun with her. I felt sad that I missed out on that with my son."

Once she had quit nursing, and with her OB's guidance and support, she started an antidepressant, at 6 months postpartum. Initially, she took Zoloft, which robbed her of emotion and made her feel like a "zombie," so she switched to Lexapro. It proved more effective for her. She encourages other mothers considering medication to remember that everyone responds differently to antidepressants, and sometimes switching is necessary. Lucy is thankful to her OB, who prompted her to check back in after she started the Zoloft, and notify the office if she had any issues with the medicine. The OB "definitely made it clear that there were many medication options out there."

Lucy is now more proactive when it comes to her own mental health, and regularly tells her story to others. She wants women to know postpartum depression exists, and to seek help sooner than she did. It's critical, she says, to understand that postpartum depression is complicated and manifests differently. It doesn't necessarily fit neatly into categories like crying spells or psychosis.

Hard Conversations

Delaying treatment—or never getting it—isn't just painful. It can be damaging to a mother and her family. Left unchecked, post-partum depression can lead to chronic depression in mothers, and interfere with mother-child bonding. Children whose mothers haven't sought treatment are more likely to develop emotional and behavioral problems, like sleeping and eating difficulties, excessive crying, attention-deficit/hyperactivity disorder (ADHD), and delays in language development (Mayo Clinic Staff, 2015). Despite the risks, some studies indicate that only 15 percent of women with postpartum depression actually get professional treatment (Tartakovsky, 2016).

That number should serve to remind us why we have to break barriers to treatment, like stigma and access to health care. Otherwise, a mother and her family could sustain permanent damage, says Katherine Stone, founder of Postpartum Progress Inc., a national nonprofit dedicated to raising awareness and providing peer support for women with maternal mental illness. Broaching the topic of PMADs with expectant mothers is key, according to Stone, because they don't think they'll get the illnesses, they're not aware of how common they are, or they don't know the risk factors: "You have childbirth-education classes where they go over it for like two minutes. They don't talk enough about it and what can happen."

Why aren't the conversations more frequent? Stone says it's partly because of how pregnant women and new mothers are perceived. "They are already so emotional. Let's not talk about anything negative and affect their psyches because they are so fragile. So we don't have the conversations." It's more beneficial to a mother in the long run if we reveal how ugly PMADs can be—not to scare her, but to empower her with knowledge. Ideally, this will help make her less afraid to seek treatment. Stone says,

> They used to put women in mental institutions and never let them out, so we've gotten past that. But there's just a lot left to do. ... I hear from women all over the world and country, and I hate hearing the stories of women who are missed by doctors or suffer way too long because they think nothing could be done. You see so much needless suffering. That's frustrating.

The Suicide Factor

In the worst cases, depressive thinking can be deadly. The risk for suicidality—which includes suicide deaths, intentional self-harm, and thoughts of death and self-harm—is significantly increased among depressed women in the perinatal period (Lindahl et al., 2005). And while the rate of completed suicide is lower in postpartum women than in the general population of women, it ranks as the second-leading cause of maternal death (Wisner et al., 2013).

The case of Cynthia Wachenheim, the 44-year-old New York lawyer who jumped to her death in March 2013, drew national attention. Her 10-month-old son was strapped to her and survived the fall. In a detailed suicide note, she blamed herself for the baby falling a few times, which she thought might have caused a health condition that would hinder him for life. She wrote about her friends, family, and pediatrician not believing her (Hartocollis & Ruderman, 2013).

"I became so low, thinking that if I had unknowingly caused brain damage to my beautiful, precious baby, I didn't want to live," she wrote. Wachenheim appeared fine until the baby was around 4 months old. She had no risk factors to suggest she might become delusional and suicidal (Belluck, 2014).

Her longtime friend, Elizabeth Nowicki, said Wachenheim would not have ended her life if she weren't gripped by mental illness. In a message on the website Above the Law, Nowicki wrote, "She was a very gentle, quiet, loving, kind woman. She was both brilliant and rational. ... [T]here is nobody who was LESS likely to kill herself and try to harm her baby, in my mind" (Lat, 2013).

As to whether Wachenheim was suffering from postpartum depression or psychosis—it's a tricky case, Kleiman says:

> [I]f you ask 10 experts, you will get 10 different answers. So I hesitate to speculate, given that I did not treat her. I will say, though, whenever there is the potential death of a baby, (as opposed to suicide with no baby harm involved), it is more likely that psychotic symptoms are involved. That can mean postpartum psychosis. It can also mean severe postpartum depression with psychotic symptoms.

Screening could hold a key to catching mood disorders sooner and preventing tragedies. Among the women in Dr. Katherine Wisner's 2013 study who screened positive for depression, 19.3 percent had thoughts about harming themselves. "Most of these women would not have been screened and therefore would not have been identified as seriously at risk," Wisner said. "We believe screening will save lives" (Paul, 2013).

One of the most successful screening tools for PPD is the Edinburgh Postpartum Depression Scale (EPDS), a 10-item questionnaire that gives women scores between 0 and 30. Most clinics using EPDS set 10 as the cutoff score, which identifies more than 90 percent of women with postpartum depression. The questionnaire focuses on psychological aspects of depression, and explores both depression and anxiety (Thurgood et al., 2009). As part of a 2004 study, a residency program used EPDS and saw detection of postpartum depression jump from 6.3 percent of identified cases to 35.4 percent. EPDS was then used as part of a community program, where detection increased from 3.7 percent to 10.7 percent (Thurgood et al., 2009). (For more on screening, see Chapter 9.)

I didn't have suicidal thoughts after Noah was born. But I did get pulled into a vortex of depressive thinking. It has the power to twist life into what seems like a pointless charade. I was fortunate to receive effective treatment, to have doctors who worked on my behalf, with whom I could have conversations well beyond my comfort zone. Not once did they suggest I was losing my mind. Along with my friends and family, they encouraged me and helped me heal.

For the pregnant or postpartum woman contending with stigma, an identity crisis, or even suicidal thoughts, proper treatment and a loving, informed community of supporters are her best line of defense. It is up to us—survivors of mood disorders, doctors, nurses, therapists, friends, and family of new mothers—to step in and spur the difficult discussions Stone mentioned. They may be uncomfortable. But they could mean the difference between life and death.

We must remind a struggling new mother that a mood disorder is a time and place that she must move through, but it doesn't define her character. When my brother reminded me of that truth, he provided a shield of hope. It protected me from the blaze of intrusive images, which I believed wouldn't end. As it turns out, Jim was right. The terrifying images were temporary. And so was my illness.

CHAPTER 7

What About Dad?

Help by and for Men

God wills that we have sorrow here,
*   And we will share it;*
Whisper thy sorrow in mine ear
*   That I may also bear it;*
If anywhere our trouble seems
*   To find an end,*
'Tis in the fairy-land of dreams,
Or with a friend.

LIONEL TENNYSON, *Sympathy*

The month after I had Noah, my mind felt like an egg frying in its own shell—a gluey orb torched by unwelcome thoughts and unfounded fears, masked only by the smoothness of skull and skin. In the fragility of those days, I wondered if something could irreparably fracture my mind. Before I started therapy and medication, I reached for help from three trustworthy sources: my husband, Matt, my family, and my friends.

I first shared my intrusive images with Matt. They were recurring thoughts of our son falling down a trash chute, a frying pan hitting him in the head, and my aversion to forks. Matt didn't have previous experience with intrusive thoughts. He could have balked. He could have reacted in fear, and taken me to the hospital for a psychiatric evaluation. But he didn't. He prayed with me. When I called my OB for more help, he supported me. When I was considering antidepressants and therapy, he helped me think through the steps, and ultimately agreed they were worth a try. Not once did I feel like he lost faith in me.

I also looked to my extended family for support, especially because my mother had died 20 years earlier (for more on this, see Chapter 1). I grieved her absence profoundly, simply because I had become a mother. Here was yet another of life's defining times, without her. The added layer of postpartum depression made me need her love and reassurance even more. Because my mother and I were emotionally close during her short life, I can guess that her mere presence would've mollified my malaise. Still, I am grateful for two people who stepped in as surrogates: my late brother, Jim, and my mother's younger sister, Linda.

Jim reminded me that my mental state was just that—a place through which I was moving. I wouldn't stay there, and it didn't define my character. That was a lifeline, tethering me to the truth that the future wouldn't be as bleak as I thought. He lived two states away, but called regularly. His love and support were unconditional.

Aunt Linda also lived out-of-state, but she came to stay with us three times. During her first visit, my crying spells reached their peak. Seeing this, and knowing it was desperately out of character for me, she came back. Each time she took care of *me*—she cooked food I wanted, brought me coffee while I nursed, and took Noah into her room and fed him several times at night, so I could sleep. She gave me prayer cards, encouraging reminders I tacked up around my apartment, and she prayed with me, reading special passages of the Bible. These unconditional tokens of love were what my own mother would have done, a veritable form of emotional gold. Aunt Linda acted as a true mother substitute, championing and loving me so I could pour love into my child.

My mother-in-law was also a source of emotional support for me, and for my husband. Our first visitor after Noah was born, she was there when my symptoms surfaced. Eventually, she helped me decide antidepressants were worth trying.

My friends were constant fixtures. Many brought or sent meals and baby gifts. We had so much food, I didn't cook dinner until Noah was more than a month old. They offered stories of their own postpartum journeys and solace. A few made special trips to stay with us and help with Noah. My email box was full of supportive notes, and my phone rang with calls of concern.

One particular band of friends, my small group from church, was like informal therapy. I conveyed to them my postpartum events as they unfolded, intrusive images and all. No one recoiled or judged. Everyone prayed and empathized.

Without these people and their generosity, I wouldn't have recovered and healed as quickly as I did. Research underscores the value of social support for new mothers, even before the baby is born. A 2013 study says pregnant women who get strong social support from their families appear to be protected from steep increases in a stress hormone released by the placenta, pCRH, which makes them less likely to develop postpartum depression

(Hahn-Holbrook et al., 2013). Dr. Christine Dunkel Schetter, a UCLA psychology professor and co-author of the study, said in a release that social support includes help with tasks, as well as emotional support—things like acceptance, listening, and making someone feel cared for and valued (Association for Psychological Science, 2013).

While researching this book, I often heard a question: "Will you include anything for husbands, so they know how to help their wives?" By design, men aren't wired to be prepared for the emotional twists and turns that await some of us in life's postpartum corridors. As my husband rightly points out, a man's inclination is to offer an immediate solution, return the family to its so-called normalcy, and move on. When it comes to perinatal mood disorders, however, fast fixes aren't the answer. A husband who tries to help might unwittingly make things worse. He needs guidance about what he should do to help his wife. He needs care and support for himself, as well. Although we tend to think of PMADs as affecting new mothers, new fathers can also fall prey to them.

I recognize the value of all social support, especially family and friends. Husbands are often the first line of defense, assuming they live with the mother and child, and they know the situation best. Yet, resources for men are scant. Seeking to fill part of the void, I have devoted this chapter to men.

Because it's easy to forget that PMADs afflict fathers, I focus first on how men experience mood disorders differently than women. I offer a real-world example of someone who lived through paternal postnatal depression, but didn't seek treatment until much later. I also include expert advice about how men can help their wives and themselves, before describing another situation in which a husband supported his wife through a prolonged ordeal with several mood disorders.

Men Get Mood Disorders Too

Mood disorders show up differently in men than they do in women. That's true during childbearing years and at other times in life. We're just starting to understand and acknowledge these differences. It is critical that we do. When a man's mental health sinks, the ripples spread to the rest of his family and may linger, especially if the illness goes untreated.

A meta-analysis published in the *Journal of the American Medical Association* (*JAMA*) says "paternal prenatal and postpartum depression has received little attention from researchers and clinicians" (Paulson & Bazemore, 2010, p. 1961). We do know a few key things, however, based on existing research. For instance, men, like women, face a higher risk of depression during pregnancy and after a child is born. The *JAMA* study examined the rates of depression among a group of 28,000 fathers, both before and after childbirth. Overall, the rate of paternal depression was 10.4 percent. Internationally, the rate was lower, at 8.2 percent. Among U.S. men, the figure was notably higher—14.1 percent (Paulson & Bazemore, 2010). Fathers had the highest rates of depression between 3 and 6 months postpartum, "although the small number of studies measuring paternal depression during this period suggests cautious interpretation" (Paulson & Bazemore, 2010, p. 1966). There was also a "moderate correlation between depression in fathers and mothers" (Paulson & Bazemore, 2010, p. 1968).

The authors say the findings have a variety of implications for how both fathers and mothers are screened and treated for PMADs:

> The observation that expecting and new fathers disproportionately experience depression suggests that more efforts should be made to improve screening and referral, particularly in light of the mounting evidence that early paternal depression may

have substantial emotional, behavioral, and developmental effects on children (Paulson & Bazemore, 2010, p. 1968).

Based on the correlation between fathers and mothers, if one parent has depression, the other should receive clinical attention: "Likewise, prevention and intervention efforts for depression in parents might be focused on the couple and family rather than the individual" (Paulson & Bazemore, 2010, p. 1968).

Depression in Men is Different

Dr. Will Courtenay, an Oakland, California-based psychotherapist and expert on men's health, says up to one in four new dads have paternal postnatal depression (PPND; Postpartum Men, n.d.). Sadly, one thing we know the least about is what puts men at risk (Postpartum Men, n.d.). While we may be looking through a glass darkly, research has shed some light on potential risk factors. They include:

- a lack of good sleep;
- a personal history of depression;
- a poor relationship with a spouse;
- a poor relationship with one or both parents;
- relationship stress with a partner or with in-laws;
- excessive stress related to becoming a parent or father;
- nonstandard family (such as being unmarried or a stepfather);
- poor social functioning;
- a lack of support from others;
- economic problems or limited resources; and
- a sense of being excluded from the connection between the mother and baby (Postpartum Men, n.d.).

Generally speaking, men with depression are more likely than women to hide their symptoms or withdraw from others, Courtenay says on his website. Not only do men experience depression differently from women, they cope in different ways. This might be part of the reason mental-health professionals frequently overlook or misdiagnose depression in men (Postpartum Men, n.d.). Courtenay cites the classic symptoms of depression, such as feeling sad, hopeless, or guilty, and a loss of interest in things, among others. He notes that men often don't acknowledge these feelings. Moreover, experts are starting to recognize symptoms unique to men. Among them are:

- increased anger and conflict with others;
- increased use of alcohol or other drugs;
- frustration or irritability;
- violent behavior;
- losing weight without trying;
- isolation from family and friends;
- being easily stressed;
- impulsiveness and taking risks, like reckless driving and extramarital sex;
- feeling discouraged;
- increases in complaints about physical problems;
- ongoing physical symptoms, like headaches, digestion problems, or pain;
- problems with concentration and motivation;
- loss of interest in work, hobbies, and sex;
- working constantly;
- misuse of prescription medication;
- increased concerns about productivity and functioning at school or work;

- fatigue;

- experiencing conflict between how you think you should be as a man and how you actually are; and

- thoughts of suicide (Postpartum Men, n.d.).

Depressed men don't have all of these symptoms. Some men encounter a few, and others deal with many. The severity changes over time and depends on the individual, Courtenay says.

Mark and Michelle: From the Trenches to Triumph

Mark Williams[20] battled a mood disorder after his son's birth in 2004, though at the time, he didn't know what to call it—and he didn't get help until years later. Mark's wife, Michelle, had a mostly uneventful pregnancy. But she spent around twenty-two hours in labor, a time he remembers as "absolutely horrendous." When the doctors explained that she needed an emergency cesarean, Mark had a panic attack, something he'd not experienced before. "I thought my wife and baby were going to die," says Mark, a native of Wales, where he lives with Michelle and their son, Ethan.

Michelle's behavior was markedly changed following the birth. She was unusually clingy, and wanted Mark to be with her at all times. Once the couple went home with Ethan, Michelle's mood worsened. Her mother, staying with them temporarily, would help take care of the baby and offer respite, but Michelle couldn't fall asleep. Her mind raced and she felt as if she were a different person. Without proper sleep for 2 weeks straight, she grew increasingly tired and unhappy, and she had trouble eating.

---

20 My personal communication with Mark Williams took place between September 15, 2015, and March 8, 2016.

She declined visitors, forced herself to eat—often gagging—and found it difficult to manage everyday tasks.

Eventually, a health visitor—a public-health nurse who works mostly with young children and their families (National Health Service, n.d.)—came to see Michelle, and suggested she might have postnatal depression (the term "postnatal" is commonly used in the UK). A community psychiatric nurse (CPN) prescribed antidepressants, which didn't help. Later, the CPN also prescribed sleeping medication. This did help Michelle sleep. But her mood was still low. She visited often with her CPNs, who grew to be like family.

Mark, who didn't know much about depression, was at first incredulous that it could steal the heart of his family. He and his wife had good jobs, a new home, the ability to buy whatever they wanted, the love and support of family and friends—all things, he figured, that should insulate them from the clutches of depression.

After a family vacation in Spain, Michelle's depression intensified. Her CPNs changed her antidepressants, which made a big difference. Michelle also started to see a psychiatrist and a psychologist. Her mother came to stay for an extended period of time, and Mark quit his job as a self-employed salesman. This allowed him to tend to household chores, Michelle, and the baby. The three of them would also spend time at his parents' home. Meanwhile, Michelle explored other paths she hoped would lead to healing: acupuncture, hypnotherapy, and a support group. She credits the group, based on cognitive therapy, as key to her recovery. After about eighteen months, she finally felt like herself.

The stress of the unexpected upheaval and a sense of isolation weighed heavily on Mark. When his son was around 6 months old, he felt lost in a fog of depression. He self-medicated with alcohol, and feelings of anger mounted. At one point, Mark, who had never before lashed out in anger, punched a sofa and broke his hand. Thoughts of suicide came to mind, though he never made a concrete plan to harm himself. He worked hard to conceal his angst from Michelle, fearing it would cause her to have setbacks with her own depression. As time went on, Michelle healed, Mark developed a strong bond with Ethan, and home life evened out.

In 2011, as Mark helped care for his grandfather stricken with dementia, his depression clawed its way back to life. Dark thoughts resurfaced, and he started drinking again. His energy flagged, and he cried frequently. Getting out of bed in the morning seemed a pointless chore. One day, he reached the end of himself and sought help. He called a local mental-health charity, which directed him to seek out his family doctor, who said he had symptoms of depression and anxiety. His doctor prescribed medication, which kicked in quickly and boosted his mood. He also started seeing a professional counselor, which was helpful from the first session.

Mark took other steps to get well. He enrolled in a mindfulness course, which lowered his stress levels, and educated himself on mental health. He focused on eating well and exercising regularly. As part of his effort to unhinge himself from stressors, he stopped working in sales, and turned instead to work in the mental-health arena. Within 7 weeks, he felt better.

While working out at the gym, Mark met another father, John, who also had postnatal depression. Standing side-by-side, the two lifted weights and shared their stories of mental anguish. John had lost his house and his business as a result of his depression, and no one had reached out to him to offer emotional support. But Mark did, and found he received as much support as he extended. It was far easier for him to open up to a stranger who had walked a similar path than it was to talk with his oldest friends. Part of this, he believes, is simply because he and John weren't face-to-face as they related their experiences. "Men talk better side-by-side," he says. Stigma also restrained Mark from being more open with people he knew well.

After he met John, he realized there was value and power in community: "[T]alking to other guys who had experienced things like me, it made me feel better as a man." Mark responded to what he learned. In 2012, he established Fathers Reaching Out, a support group for men whose wives suffer from perinatal mood and anxiety disorders, or who have mood disorders themselves.

In 2015, Mark launched another resource: Dads Matter UK, a charity designed to help fathers with depression, anxiety, and post-traumatic stress disorder. Mark started the charity along with another

> *Remember, depression is an illness, and we must treat it as [an] illness before it gets worse.*
>
> MARK WILLIAMS,
> a UK-based mental-health advocate who specializes in helping fathers

father and mental-health advocate, Chris Bingley. Chris's wife, Joanne, developed severe postpartum depression after the birth of their daughter in 2010, but didn't receive proper care and treatment. When their baby was 10 weeks old, Joanne ended her life. Chris has dedicated his life's work to mental-health issues for parents and children. Since then, Mark has left his positions at both Fathers Reaching Out and Dads Matter UK, and now runs advocacy campaigns for mental health, including workshops and talks.

Reaching Out

When Mark first launched Fathers Reaching Out, he met derisive laughter from some who didn't believe men could get perinatal mood disorders. Since then, he's encountered hundreds of fathers who, on hearing his story, divulge their own struggles—which abound. Men whose wives have difficult births or deliver still born children often harbor post-traumatic stress, and express feelings of pain and anger.

If their wives develop mood disorders, husbands sometimes get caught in their own webs of illness. They might have anxiety due to fears they won't be good fathers. If their own fathers fell short, they may feel they don't have strong role models, or that they're inclined to repeat family history. Some new mothers take a break from or quit their jobs, which can stir new financial concerns for fathers. Among the men Mark has met, some "were working in jobs they hated and having anxiety about that, and they felt trapped in needing to support a family."

Managing such stress can be messy business. "Unfortunately, men tend to use negative coping skills like drinks or anger. Even domestic violence has come up, as well," Mark says. Depression may manifest in self-harm, overspending, and overworking. "The dads who do [overwork] tend to work more because they don't want to go back to the house, where things are bad." He has helped men who turn to drugs for the first time in their lives, because they want relief.

When he speaks to struggling fathers, Mark urges them to get assistance: "It's an illness like any other illness, and the quicker you get the help, the quicker you get the recovery." Allowing it to fester invites trouble, and can lead to impaired bonding between a father and his child. He uses the analogy of the oxygen-mask instructions offered by airline flight attendants: If you're in a crisis and you don't first get help for yourself, you won't be able to help the child. He reminds men that just as their physical bodies need a break from working out, so their minds need respite, especially when a mood disorder is in the mix. They can find this mental break through a variety of outlets, such as mindfulness courses, therapy, exercise, and a healthy diet.

One of Mark's goals is to develop a clearer pathway in the UK for treating and caring for new or soon-to-be fathers with a history of mental illness. These men are likelier to develop perinatal mood disorders because of their history. He believes clinicians should screen such high-risk groups through questionnaires, and counsel them on the chances of a stressful event like childbirth taking a toll on their mental health. Because men talk more freely when they stand side-by-side, support groups should be based on this principle, and offer activities such as sports and hobbies where men aren't required to be face-to-face.

He also works to increase support for fathers who see their wives endure a difficult birth or a birth-related trauma. Watching a loved one confront something traumatic has a residual effect that often goes unnoticed, and can lead to post-traumatic stress. There isn't enough discussion about how this might impact men. "I want there to be awareness that there's a father in the room," he says.

The need for more mother-and-baby units (MBUs) is another area where Mark is raising awareness. MBUs are inpatient care facilities specifically for mothers with severe PMADs and their babies. He has witnessed women with severe mental illness who are hospitalized *without* their children, which leads to more problems: "They come out more traumatized than when they went in. The mother should be in there with a child." One woman he spoke with was in a psychiatric hospital for the first 3 years of her baby's life. "We need the proper specialists [to care for these mothers] and perinatal mental health support."

The UK has 17 mother-and-baby units (MBUs), including 15 in England and two in Scotland (Maternal Mental Health Alliance, n.d.). To date, Wales and Northern Ireland don't have any. They are operated by the publicly funded health care system, the National Health Service (NHS). These facilities provide individualized care and treatment for mothers and assist with the care of the babies. Mark isn't the only one who thinks it's critical to have more MBUs. In January 2016, former British Prime Minister David Cameron pledged £290 million to be used for additional beds in the MBUs, and to create new community perinatal mental health teams (Campbell, 2016). The United States, by comparison, has just three inpatient units, in North Carolina, California, and New York—but none of them allow babies to stay overnight. Dr. Wendy Davis, executive director of Postpartum Support International, points out, "There are several intensive outpatient programs that include babies, but we need more! We are definitely behind the UK, New Zealand and Australia." (See Chapter 9 for more on mother-baby units and inpatient care facilities for new mothers.)

Helping You, Helping Me

Mark's personal experiences and his work in the mental-health arena have equipped him with a knowledge of how men can help themselves and their wives. Men must prioritize their mental health after childbirth, especially if their wives are struggling. "Looking after yourself is most important, [because] if you're unwell, the family's well-being can suffer, too. Exercise and healthy eating help," he says.

He urges men to work at bonding with their babies, even if it's difficult. Taking family walks is an excellent way of doing that, and it can boost mental health. Above all, if a father has an unshakable sense something is wrong, he should seek professional help. For those concerned about taking medication, he reminds them it's generally a temporary remedy to return them to full health: "Remember, depression is an illness, and we must treat it as [an] illness before it gets worse."

To help their wives, men should first educate themselves on perinatal mood disorders and contact a health professional for guidance. "As the partner, I would reduce stress as much as you can in other parts of your life," he says. You can do this through relaxation and positive coping skills, such as mindfulness. It's wise to avoid moving or changes in employment, if possible, as well as alcohol and drugs. "Make sure you're offloading your worries to either a counselor or someone who knows about mental health, possibly a friend." Support groups for new fathers can be a valuable place to share your concerns and learn from peers.

What Dads Can Do

Someone else who has made a dent in the dearth of information geared to husbands is postpartum expert Karen Kleiman. Her book, *The Postpartum Husband: Practical Solutions for Living with Postpartum Depression*, helps readers understand and identify mood disorders, and covers topics such as coping, treatment options, and common feelings men contend with, including worry, anger, and confusion.

A more concise resource is a chapter for husbands in the book Kleiman co-authored with Dr. Valerie Davis Raskin, *This Isn't What I Expected: Overcoming Postpartum Depression*. The chapter educates men on the symptoms their wives might exhibit, how they can help their wives and themselves, and includes a husband's retelling of his wife's two encounters with postpartum depression. Kleiman and Raskin offer a host of things a husband can do to help his wife:

▶ **Listen and validate.** Be available to hear how she's feeling, even if she repeats herself. Remind her that your support is unwavering: "Your instincts about what to do may not work, or may actually increase the emotional distance between the two of you. For example, responding to her distress with logic or advice, or trying to be firm with her, may not be effective, because they may make her feel misunderstood or alienated from you."

▶ **Try to be patient.** The most grueling days with a mood disorder seem to last forever, but recovery does come, albeit gradually: "We see many fathers who, once the PPD is identified, feel compelled to 'fix' it. It is perfectly understandable that you both want this to go away immediately. Unfortunately, there are no quick fixes or magic spells to ease the pain."

▸ **Give her breaks.** Help your wife reserve time for rest, relaxation, or indulging in a pleasure. Don't assume she'll ask for help, so get comfortable making regular offers, such as picking up dinner on the way home or doing laundry.

▸ **Give her the okay to be less interested in sex.** Most women afflicted with postpartum depression aren't interested in sex. Don't take it personally. Keep communication lines open when it comes to intimacy, and reassure your wife that you won't stray or leave her.

▸ **Offer emotional support.** Saying supportive things can be tricky, because PPD brings extra sensitivity. A few things to try: Tell her you love her; remind her you're glad she's the mother of your child; be sensitive to how she feels about her body; and tell her she's pretty.

▸ **Back her decision to get help in the form of individual therapy, medication, support groups, or otherwise.** Being a source of encouragement, gathering information as she takes different steps, finding ways to manage treatment costs instead of dwelling on them—these are helpful.

▸ **Look for signs of an emergency.** "If you think that your wife or the baby is in danger, you must override her decision to avoid treatment. Someone who is at risk of hurting herself or hurting someone else can be legally forced to receive treatment and/ or hospitalization." It's scary but rare. Some red flags include talk of hurting herself or the baby; hallucinations; extreme, persistent hopelessness; and self-destructive behaviors (Kleiman & Raskin, 2013, pp. 203-224).

Just as critical as caring for your wife, Kleiman and Raskin say, is taking care of yourself. Here are some ways to do just that:

- **Give yourself credit.** If your wife has a PMAD, you will likely have added responsibilities at home and with the baby, on top of your day job, where you might feel extra pressure now that you're providing for a family. When you add all of this to sleep deprivation, it can stir up the worst time in life: "Give yourself a pat on the back before you do anything else, because it may be a while before anyone else recognizes what a wonderful job you are doing."

- **Talk with someone you trust.** Finding a safe haven for conversation is key, because "talking is absolutely the most underrated way to manage this emotional assault." Consider close friends, family members, other new fathers, a support group if it's available, or a therapist.

- **Take care of yourself.** This means exercising, eating, and sleeping well and resting, and staying in touch with friends.

- **If your wife complains, try not to take it to heart.** A woman with a mood disorder is often hypercritical—something that fades with recovery.

- **Let yourself have negative feelings.** Feeling cheated, angry and/or fearful is a reasonable response to the mayhem introduced by a mood disorder. Instead of trying to contain the emotions, admit you have them, educate yourself about PMADs, and take steps to get help for yourself and your wife (Kleiman & Raskin, 2013, pp. 203-224).

For more information, see the Resources section at the back of this book.

David and Jill: Finding Their Way Together

The darkness of depression all but devoured the woman David Denton's wife, Jill,[21] once was. It was the last thing either of them expected. "My wife has wanted to have kids her whole life. We met at an orphanage in India [while on a missions trip]. She has a deep love for kids," David says. They tried to have children as soon as they got married, but Jill had a miscarriage. She later was diagnosed with polycystic ovarian syndrome. It was 9 years and a lot of heartache before she got pregnant with their daughter.

> We are grounded in our faith and we know God is sovereign, and we know he is in control. Even though we believe that, it [was] hard to watch others get pregnant. When we got pregnant, it was a long-awaited expectation.

Going into the pregnancy, Jill "was pumped," and they began to believe their worries about miscarriage were over. Still, cautious optimism had them wait to share the news with friends and family until they reached the 3-month mark.

They took 7 weeks of classes on natural childbirth. Jill wanted to labor mostly at home and head to the hospital when birth was imminent. An epidural was not part of their plan. When she went into labor, their plans were dashed. Jill's water broke, and doctors summoned them to the hospital immediately. There, her labor didn't progress, and she was induced. David says,

> She tried to labor as much as she could, but physically, she couldn't do it, so she opted for the epidural. All the natural-childbirth-class stuff started crumbling. I didn't have any expectations. I was just glad to have a baby. If we labored at home or at the

---

21 My personal communication with Jill and David Denton took place between September 14, 2015, and February 25, 2016.

hospital, there was no problem there. But for her, it was a major deal.

Nursing was also important to Jill. But the baby wouldn't latch properly and didn't get ample milk, which led to her not sleeping well. They realized that their child wasn't eating enough, so David and Jill switched from nursing to bottle-feeding. Again, this didn't bother David. He simply wanted his child to eat and sleep well. It was different for Jill. She believed nursing was a critical part of being a good mother. Seeing others around her who had no trouble nursing made it even more difficult.

Jill wasn't eating or sleeping much, and she fell into fits of uncontrollable tears. "My wife is not an emotional person to begin with. Going into the third or fourth week, I knew something wasn't right. She'd be crying hysterically," David says. On her personal blog, Jill details her experience:

> Then I found myself absolutely HATING to be alone at home with the baby. I would panic. This awful sick feeling would come in my stomach and a burning sensation across my back. I started calling my husband at work a lot and would just cry. I had no clear explanation for my crying. My baby was not doing anything that would cause a mom to feel upset. She ate, she slept, she loved being held, she loved her swing...overall she was a pretty content baby, but for some reason I just COULD NOT feel at peace (Denton, 2013).

She was in a constant state of fear, worried if the baby broke out crying, she would be unable to console her. Jill dreaded being at home, so the family often went out in public, where she felt disconnected, as if she were "floating around in a bubble." A spool of racing thoughts and mounting anxiety rendered her unable to focus on anything, including eating and sleeping. David, a music and youth pastor at a church near their home in Arkansas, approached his boss, who offered empathy and suggested he work from home. "I know a lot of guys aren't able to do this," David says. It "was huge because while the baby slept, I'd work on stuff, and be with my family the rest of the time."

At her 6-week postpartum checkup, Jill explained the symptoms of anxiety and depression to her OB/GYN, who gave her a low-dose prescription for an antidepressant. It gave her hope. Finally, she thought, something to help lift her from the quagmire. But the darkness lingered. A nonstop spiral of panic attacks and intrusive images overwhelmed her. Jill writes,

> If I was around her [the baby] my mind was so disturbed. Although when I was away from her the feelings of depression were paralyzing. I could not handle being around the baby, but I also couldn't handle being away from her. I was so trapped (Denton, 2013).

As a last resort, Jill separated from her daughter. She went to stay with her parents, who live nearby, for 6 weeks. She started to see a therapist and a psychiatrist, and changed medications. When she felt stable enough to visit David and the baby, she took specific medication so she could try to reap a bit of enjoyment from the experience. Though some of her symptoms improved, others intensified. David says it was as if common sense had been dashed from Jill's radar when it came to caring for their daughter.

My husband is incredible. He was my rock during these days. He did not shy away from the problem at hand. Instead, he took hold of it and did everything in his power to fight for me.

JILL DENTON,
explaining how her husband,
David, helped her recover

Soon, she battled daily thoughts of suicide. Reaching the end of herself, she packed her bags and planned to leave town. Instead, she ended up at the public library, where she landed on information about the Perinatal Psychiatry Inpatient Unit at the University of North Carolina's Center for Women's Mood Disorders in Chapel Hill, N.C. Instinct told her it was a place worth pursuing, and David agreed. With the help of her psychiatrist, Jill applied to the program and was accepted. Along with David, the baby, and her mother, Jill drove to North Carolina. She was admitted on a Friday. By Sunday, she was improving.

Ultimately diagnosed with postpartum depression and anxiety disorders, postpartum OCD, and panic disorder, Jill says a combination of factors led to her recovery. The doctors at UNC changed her medications and increased the dosages, and gave her medication to help her sleep. "Within the first 48 hours I noticed a huge difference," she said in an email exchange.

> The nursing staff was incredibly attentive, and there was something about their gentle, understanding approach that aided my healing. I received both one-on-one and group therapy, and in those times, I learned valuable coping tools to help control my racing thoughts (J. Denton, personal communication, February 23, 2016).

She met individually with several doctors, whose care she calls "life-changing." They taught her about the illness she was fighting, and how to cope with it. Meanwhile, the medication took effect and enabled her to put the coping mechanisms to work. David and the baby visited her for long periods of time. As soon as she felt like herself again, caring for and bonding with the baby came naturally to her. "I know that's not the case for all women, so I'm thankful I had that," she says.

The UNC facility is one of three perinatal psychiatric inpatient programs in the United States. It offers individualized treatment for patients battling severe PMADs, including management of medication, occupational and recreational therapy, spiritual and nutritional counseling, and education, which includes support for family members. If a mother is struggling with how to care for her newborn, the program can help her. Extended visiting hours maximize mother-baby interaction and bonding. (For more on inpatient programs in the United States and the UK, see Chapter 9.) "For my wife, getting her to that facility was a life-changer," David says.

"Be a Detective"

Based on what he's learned, David seeks now to help other new fathers. Above all, he encourages them to get involved as much as possible with their wives' illnesses, and to fully investigate the situation, like a detective. That means starting at the source, and noticing the wife's behavior, especially when it comes to eating and sleeping. It's a red flag if she can't do either or both. "Those two are the absolute clearest signs to me now. But I didn't know it at the time, that they're clear signs of postpartum [depression]. That'd be good for the moms and dads to know," he says. Taking stock of her emotional state of mind also matters. If, like Jill, she doesn't have a history of crying easily, but after childbirth she's suddenly crying without cause, this is reason for concern.

Once the husband has a sense of what might be going on with his wife, he should ask questions beyond the confines of home. That means chasing down people in the medical community. "Even though my wife didn't share a lot of things, I figured out why she was crying. It's like being a detective: calling nurses and getting information, etc." David, who grew up with only brothers, entered fatherhood with a limited knowledge of how the female body and mind work. Still, he pressed on, calling doctors and nurses on the weekends and after hours. "I was asking questions because I thought there was something wrong with my wife." If a doctor didn't return his call, David kept calling until he got an answer.

This strategy isn't necessarily second nature for men, though. That could be even truer when a man's family life is upended by disorder, the usual kind brought on by a newborn, and the less-usual kind that comes with mood disorders. The stress can seem uncontrollable. David has met men who haven't even considered doing detective work on behalf of their wives' mental health: "My mentality is getting in there and getting it done. But I think guys need to step up to the plate, and if they can't figure it out, get some help." Getting help is key. A man shouldn't assume his wife will seek it on her own. He says,

> She's an emotional wreck and she needs an advocate to take care of her, and to walk with her through it. And not just get home from work and sit on the couch and watch football the rest of the afternoon.

David acknowledges that they were graced with the help of Jill's parents and his understanding boss. Not everyone is as fortunate. Still, he says, he would've quit his job if it meant preserving his family: "I know it maybe sounds foolish. But my wife comes first."

A selfless man who champions his wife's cause is invaluable. Jill attests to this on her blog, where she discusses David's role in her illness and recovery:

> My husband is incredible. He was my rock during these days. He did not shy away from the problem at hand. Instead, he took hold of it and did everything in his power to fight for me. He called my doctors, he drove me to appointments. He asked questions. He gathered information. He prayed. He prayed. He prayed. He took a leave of absence from work and stayed home and took care of our baby night and day. He kept telling me over and over that he was not going to let me stay in that condition and that he was going to do whatever he had

to in order for me to get well. He loved me through the sickness. I am so grateful for his strength, love, and dedication (Denton, 2013).

If David knew then what he knows now, he would have acted faster in getting Jill to the UNC program. He didn't know it existed until she found it at the library. This underscores the dearth of helpful information out there for new fathers when it comes to maternal mental health. Closing that knowledge gap is vital. It means better education is needed for parents-to-be, and for OB/GYNs. David believes OBs ought to be required to share a brochure with expectant parents. It should have clear, succinct language about the symptoms of PMADs—such as insomnia, an inability to eat, crying spells, and trouble bonding with the baby—and what to do if they arise. It's important for doctors to be aware of inpatient programs like UNC, and refer patients to them when necessary. One of Jill's first calls for help was to her OB, who suggested she likely had the baby blues, and that her symptoms were normal.

How Birth Trauma Affects Men

When I was born in 1974, my dad didn't join my mom in the delivery room. When I asked him why not, he said, with a wave of his hand, that he saw as much as he wanted to: a healthy baby carried out to him, clucking and cooing. He didn't feel he'd missed anything by not bearing witness to the mess of childbirth. Once I had my own children, I wondered if my dad took the easy way. Didn't he let my mom do the hard part, and seek only to share in the revelry of the reward? That may be only half-true. Dr. Judith Walzer Leavitt, author of *Make Room for Daddy: The Journey From Waiting Room to Birthing Room*, says,

> During the 1960s, most hospitals, under pressure from birthing women, laymen, the women's

movement, and childbirth reform groups, admitted men into labor rooms, but not until the 1970s—and in some hospitals the 1980s—were the doors to the delivery room open to men. Beginning in the 1980s, men have felt enormous pressure to be with their wives throughout the birth process (University of North Carolina Press, n.d.).

Maybe my dad wasn't allowed into the room where I was born—on interviewing him, he said he couldn't recall the hospital's policy. Whatever the case, he was protected from potentially unsettling sights, which he'd never be able to unsee. Bringing a human being into the world is, after all, a violent act.

Remarkable and beautiful as it is, childbirth is difficult, messy, and violent by necessity. Even in the best circumstances, where no trauma comes to the mother or baby, the impression left on those witnessing childbirth is indelible, especially for first-time fathers. Those who do witness a traumatic birth could be at higher risk for PTSD. Along these lines, researchers and advocates in the UK have called for increased resources and support systems for fathers present during traumatic births, and for paternal mental health overall. Mark Williams, for example, campaigns for more counseling of fathers during pregnancy. Do they have a history of mental-health issues themselves? That's important to know, Mark says, because it means they're more vulnerable to a recurrence once the baby comes along. Someone should also explain to fathers what sorts of emergencies might crop up during the birth, so they're better prepared. When a traumatic event transpires in childbirth, Mark says, "A lot of dads keep it in, their feelings, trying to be strong for the mother, and deep down, they are suffering."

We need increased mental-health resources for new fathers—and men in general—in the United States too. I've seen first-hand how depression can manifest in a man. My brother fell into a severe depression in his mid-40s, and he ended his life. As Dr. Courtenay rightly suggests, mood disorders present differently in men than they do in women. I tried to pull on my postpartum experience to help my brother. Some of the same rules applied, but most didn't. His battle was quite different from mine. What I understand now is that he masked his symptoms for longer than I knew, largely because he didn't want to ask for help. He was an alpha-male, used to being the strong provider and helper. Admitting weakness didn't come naturally to him. When he did seek help, he didn't find a place where, or a person with whom, he felt comfortable and fully understood. Part of that was a failing of our mental-health system.

Improving Mental Health Care

We can do better for our men, and for our families. One way is through improved mental-health screening. When a woman gets pregnant, both she and her partner should take an assessment, and speak with a trained therapist about any concerns, or personal or family history of mood disorders. Waiting until the baby arrives is too late.

In addition to screening, we need better education and exchanges of information between caregivers and expectant parents. Both mothers and fathers should be involved in these talks. At some point during the pregnancy, they ought to receive information on birth trauma and perinatal mood disorders. This isn't to instill fear. It would help them understand what can go wrong during childbirth, such as an emergency C-section after a prolonged attempt at a vaginal birth, or a forceps delivery leading to an injury in the mother. It would provide an overview of the different PMADs, and emphasize that they're temporary, treatable illnesses. Discussing the stigma surrounding mental illness is fundamental, because stigma keeps many from getting help. Seeking help isn't a sign of weakness or failure. It's a strong step toward mental health for the whole family, and caregivers would do well to remind parents of that.

Part of the information shared with parents should be a list of local resources, including support groups and therapists who specialize in PMADs, books, and websites. OB/GYN offices can point parents to national groups, particularly Postpartum Support International, and the three perinatal psychiatric inpatient programs. (For more on these, see Chapter 9.) OBs need to be able and willing to help patients get in touch with these valuable resources, if the need arises.

As the *JAMA* study on depression in new fathers suggests, if one parent develops a perinatal mood disorder, the other should be monitored. Care has to be administered with an eye on keeping the *entire* family healthy, not just the person showing signs of an illness. A family's mental health is delicately intertwined. When one member hurts, everyone else does too. Research shows that when a parent is in poor mental health, the child suffers.

Untreated mental illness can show up later in life, as it did for Mark Williams. Triggered by something else, his illness packed an even stronger punch the second time around. If a parent doesn't confront and seek treatment for his illness—or if he dies by suicide—the result can be like an earthquake with never-ending aftershocks. They might show up in a child's life unexpectedly, even in adulthood. John, the friend Mark made at the gym, was in his 20s when he lost his father to suicide. John didn't address the trauma he endured as a result of his father's suicide and death. He was jolted by the emotional turmoil, but not until he became a father for the third time, in his early 40s, and his wife was battling postnatal depression. "All the stuff came back because he hadn't dealt with issues around his father," Mark says.

After I lost my brother to suicide, I realized that he had shown signs of depression and anxiety years before he admitted to struggling. I overlooked the signs, partly because I didn't recognize them as such, and because he seemed an unlikely candidate for mental illness. Jim may not have considered them as symptoms of an illness either. Still, he waited too long to get professional help. His level of desperation was difficult to treat, despite the shortcomings of the system treating him. A friend of mine who's a clinical psychologist says there is a type of depression so resistant to treatment, it's similar to advanced cancer: not hopeless, but incredibly challenging. Waiting until the 11th hour to confront any illness, physical or mental, is bad practice. Some in the breast-cancer-prevention world, encouraging women to be vigilant about their health, have coined a phrase, "Early Detection Saves Lives." Likewise, we in the mental-health community can confidently say that early detection of mood disorders saves families and lives.

CHAPTER 8

A Struggle Worth Sharing

How Women Heal From PMADs

But more often than not, the most healing thing that we can do with someone who is in pain, rather than trying to get rid of that pain, is to sit there and be willing to share it. We have to learn to hear and to bear other people's pain.

M. Scott Peck,

Further Along the Road Less Traveled

My postpartum journey rendered me like Curious George. Darting from the safe confines of home, he ambled lost in the big city, wound up in a tangle of spaghetti, and was tear-soaked after a fall broke his leg. Similar to George, I found myself confused and broken. I needed fixing.

Until I became a mother, I thought I had cool control over my emotions. I trusted my feelings as truth. I didn't understand how they had become so tangled after having a baby, why I couldn't willfully stop the tears and intrusive images, or at least ignore them. But it dawned on me that feelings can be fickle and untrue. Some of mine, for instance, suggested that God had made a mistake in letting me have a child, and that I was incapable of being a good mother. I didn't know it then, but I was on the verge of a journey that would change me, perhaps more than any other. It was a journey toward healing—something I'm still doing to this day.

This chapter deals with healing, and the strategies mothers use to pursue it physically and mentally. In the first part, I highlight what worked for me, and what I would've done differently. The rest of the chapter focuses on the stories of two other mothers and how they healed.

We can't overcome PMADs in our own power. We need to admit our weakness and ask for help. That help fortifies us as it carries us along a path toward healing. We start to recognize ourselves not as women worn out by maladies, but as new-and-stronger versions of ourselves, permanently changed by our journeys. Rife as they are with trauma, pain, and heartache, they bring us closer to the women God intends us to be. They are valuable.

If we share our stories, one of the first discoveries we make is how sharing helps us heal. Soon, others respond. We meet fellow parents contending with PMADs, or people who've battled mental illness outside the postpartum window, like men with lifelong depression. Our willingness to reveal our struggles helps them heal, too. We recount how wrenching our days have been with as much fervor as when we relate our triumphs. We do this knowing that one day our children will be heartened by our histories of good *and* bad. Our gift to them is a legacy of strength and courage for life's hard days, weeks, and years.

Postpartum, we are so vulnerable. There has to be room in that path and that vulnerable, tender, bewildering time to be given an opportunity to advocate for our own health and our own journey back to ourselves. While we are extremely vulnerable, we are extremely fierce, and that can't be lost.

MELISSA BANGS,
who battled postpartum psychosis
after the birth of her daughter

What Worked for Me: Acting Fast, Therapy, and a Thyroid Fix

Although I didn't lose my hold on reality, I worried that I might, especially if I waited too long to seek help. What enabled me to overcome my illness was a mix of ingredients: talking to friends and family, prayers, sleep, calling my doctor quickly, antidepressants, therapy, and thyroid medication.

When the cascade of intrusive thoughts started to fall, it only took a few days for me to share them with my husband. I asked for prayers from those I trusted, and I worked on my relationship with God. This took some doing. I had what I'd call a partial Christian faith. My life was blown apart at age 15, when my mother died from breast cancer. It left me with a lingering suspicion of God. I still fight doubts that He is after my best interests. From the time I was a teenager, I have lived in self-protection mode. My postpartum experience challenged these entrenched thoughts and behaviors, and afforded me a chance to get to know God better. It's a lifelong pursuit. (For more on this, see Chapters 1 and 10.)

I also focused on getting sleep. Time has showed me that I need at least 8 or 9 hours a night. Running on the inevitable fumes of new-parent sleep loss would leave me especially light-headed, lethargic, and mind-muddled. So I pieced together shut-eye out of whatever time I could. I asked visitors and my husband to take night-feeding shifts when possible, napping when my son napped. (For more on sleep, see the side-bar in this chapter, "What Interrupted Sleep Means for New Parents.")

These efforts helped, but I was still uncomfortable in my own skin. Until I reached out to my OB/GYN, I felt as if I were swimming through pea soup, my ankles shackled by boulders. But now I know I acted rather fast. It turned out to be a saving grace, God's way of using my usual impatience for my own good. If I had delayed, I might've gotten worse. In most cases, perinatal mood disorders don't simply vanish on their own. We don't get beyond them by grinning and bearing the trouble, or because we adopt a more positive approach to life. We need help from others—doctors, therapists, family, and friends. We should be allowed to ask for such help without worrying about judgment, from ourselves or from others.

Under my OB's care, I started taking 50 milligrams (mg) of sertraline each day for 2 weeks. At that point, she said, I should double the dose, to 100 mg a day. Within 10 days, the crying spells ended and the intrusive thoughts lessened. I was wrong. My brain wasn't beyond repair, and the medication was helpful.

I stayed on it for 4 months, and during that time, I met once a week with my therapist, Rachel. She used supportive therapy, which is conversation-based, and relies on praise, advice, clarification, confrontation, and interpretation to help a patient gain understanding. (For more on different therapies, see Chapter 3.)

My sessions with Rachel helped in several ways. They let me come to terms with the reality that becoming a mother would stir up residual grief from losing my own mother 20 years earlier. (For more on this, see Chapter 1.) They also allowed me to confront and interpret the major driver of my illness: Because of birth trauma, I was mourning a loss of my expectations—things didn't go according to my plan. I felt like a failure. Rachel offered healthy strategies for reflecting on the trauma and integrating it into my life. She also pointed out that while I didn't have my own mother, it was okay to lean on other women as mother figures. In time, I came to see I hadn't failed. I did the best I could, with the resources and situations at hand.

Above all, therapy was a place for me to share my postpartum story, and to be understood. As PMAD expert Dr. Diana Barnes points out in Chapter 3, simply diagnosing a patient and treating the symptoms can lead to improvements. But deeper healing and more fundamental changes happen when the therapist understands what's behind the woman's illness.

The one-two punch of medication and therapy helped knock out many of my symptoms. But it didn't address a key issue, which was something I believe was at the root of my trouble from the beginning: an autoimmune disorder.

An Autoimmune Surprise

A few months after I stopped the medication and therapy, I learned that I had developed Hashimoto's disease, an autoimmune disorder characterized by an imbalanced thyroid (for more on this, see Chapter 1). To supplement my lack of hormones, at first I took Synthroid. When I became pregnant with my daughter, my endocrinologist increased my Synthroid dose to protect her health, and mine. An unborn child's thyroid gland isn't fully functional until after 12 weeks of pregnancy; without enough thyroid hormones, the odds of a miscarriage are greater, and the baby faces a higher risk of developmental problems (Shomon, 2017).

My thyroid problem was diagnosed 7 years ago. Taking Synthroid helped for a while, and blood tests showed my hormone levels within range, which satisfied my endocrinologist. When I mentioned other symptoms, and that Synthroid was no longer effective for me, she refused to prescribe an alternative. So, I looked for a different caregiver. I now see a physician assistant, who is progressive in her approach and has allowed me to try more natural medications, such as Armour Thyroid and Nature-Throid. I also see a chiropractor who practices applied kinesiology, a system that evaluates structural, chemical, and mental aspects of health through manual muscle testing (International College of Applied Kinesiology-USA, n.d.). My chiropractor regularly tests both my thyroid and pituitary glands. He treats me based on what he finds, and sometimes prescribes supplements. I've also altered my eating habits and I exercise regularly. If I find someone who has Hashimoto's disease, I compare notes—that's how I found my current caregivers. These extra measures greatly improve my quality of life. Living with Hashimoto's is like tending a garden; if I don't keep up, weeds grow.

A one-pill-cures-all remedy doesn't exist for Hashimoto's, so it's best to be aware of different treatments and options available, and try new things. If one route doesn't yield results, another will.

I'm convinced my thyroid imbalance was one driver of my postpartum chaos. I don't have scientific proof, in the form of a blood test. My OB didn't think I fit the profile of someone with Hashimoto's, so I don't know what my hormone levels were in those first days after Noah was born. I do know my body, though. I know it didn't feel fully well until we addressed the thyroid issue. My current doctors and a number of experts I've interviewed agree it's essential to test a new mother's thyroid levels, whether or not she shows signs of a mood disorder.

What Interrupted Sleep Means for New Parents

When I was pregnant with Noah, I often heard from others—long-time friends, people who were already parents, strangers on the street—that I should brace for a sleepless life. They didn't elaborate on the concept of interrupted sleep. That's what most new parents contend with, stirring multiple times a night to feed their newborns. A study by researchers at Tel Aviv University in Israel found that interrupted sleep has an injurious impact on mood and sustained attention (Kahn et al., 2014).

Researcher Avi Sadeh says night wakings as short as 5 to 10 minutes disrupt the natural rhythm of sleep, particularly in parents and doctors on call: "The impact of such night wakings on an individual's daytime alertness, mood, and cognitive abilities had never been studied. Our study is the first to demonstrate seriously deleterious cognitive and emotional effects" (Tel Aviv University, 2014).

The study examined the impact of sleep loss on a group of student volunteers. Their attention and self-reported moods were tested at two different times—after a normal, 8-hour night of sleep, and after a night of either reduced or interrupted sleep. Participants in the reduced-sleep group had only 4 hours straight, while those in the interrupted-sleep group were roused four times across 8 hours of slumber (Kahn et al., 2014). Compared to the normal night of sleep, the nights of both reduced and interrupted sleep led to problems with attention, and an increase in depression, fatigue, and confusion levels, and reduced vigor (Kahn et al., 2014). According to Sadeh,

> Our study shows the impact of only one disrupted night. But we know that these effects accumulate and therefore the functional price new parents— who awaken three to ten times a night for months

on end—pay for common infant sleep disturbance
is enormous (Tel Aviv University, 2014).

Dr. Christina Hibbert, an Arizona-based clinical psychologist
and expert on maternal mental health, echoes those findings.
She says sleep loss is associated with a variety of emotional symptoms, including depression, anxiety, mood swings, irritability,
anger, frustration, and poor coping skills (Hibbert, n.d.). At the
most extreme, sleep deprivation can trigger psychotic symptoms.
Hibbert says healthy functioning in an adult requires at least 5
hours of uninterrupted sleep every 24 hours (n.d.). That's a tall
order for new parents. But without enough sleep, they face height-
ened risks for developing physical and mental-health symptoms.

Finding more sleep in those foggy first days of parenthood
may seem a more-than-formidable feat. That's especially true in in
our wired world, where everything and everyone are expected to
be accessible at all times. But it's not impossible. Hibbert suggests
new parents make sleep a priority, and establish a routine they
stick to, one that includes frequent naps and a bedtime goal.
Some of her other pointers include treating insomnia, seeking
sleep therapy when necessary, and using strategies to improve
infant sleep (Hibbert, n.d.).

Donna Rigert,[22] a birth-doula in the Chicago area, addresses
postpartum sleep deprivation with her clients. She tells them—
especially first-time mothers learning to nurse—that on arriving
home, they should retreat to their bedrooms with their babies for
24 hours, and figure out nursing in private. "You go to bed, and you
really keep the visitors at bay. You are learning how to work your
breast into another human being's mouth. You don't want to do
that in front of anyone else," Rigert says. She points women to an
article by Gloria Lemay, a birth attendant and midwife educator,

---

22   My personal communication with Donna Rigert took place between May 8, 2015,
and May 19, 2015.

which discusses this concept of rest, a so-called "babymoon" (2009). Lemay writes,

> For building up milk production, go to bed with the baby for 24 hours. Mother should wear only panties, baby only a diaper. A tray with fluids, magazines and flowers beside the bed for the mother and all diaper changing needs for the baby close at hand. Another adult woman in the house brings meals to the mother. After 24 hours of this bed rest, the milk will be abundant (2009).

In addition to nursing ills, Lemay says, bedrest can cure postpartum bleeding and "general crabbiness or depression." She encourages mothers to take their first days and weeks after childbirth slowly:

> We need to give up the notion of supermom. Do whatever it takes to get your rest time after the birth and then you will be back to your busy life sooner. ... The really smart women don't even get dressed for weeks after the birth. If you're all perky in a track suit, people will expect you to run ... therefore, find the nastiest old nightie possible and wear that to convince family and friends that you need their assistance (Lemay, 2009).

Different Roads to Wellness

While researching this book, I gained a new appreciation for my postpartum experience, both for what it was, and what it wasn't. In many respects, I was fortunate. I acted quickly and didn't give my illness a chance to mushroom. Some women aren't able to do so. They're held back by stigma, or unaware they're fighting a treatable, curable illness. In other cases, family and friends discourage them from seeking help.

My therapy and medication worked well for my mind and body. That's not true in each case. Sometimes it's necessary to switch medication several times, or find a different therapist.

If I knew then what I know now, I'd have done a few things differently. I would've asked my OB to order a thyroid blood test the week after Noah was born. Even if the eventual dysfunction didn't surface right away, at least I would have known what my hormones were doing. I also would've explored natural remedies, such as those offered by my current chiropractor, and used them to bolster the work of my therapist and the antidepressant. A woman should have knowledge of the different tools at her disposal. These days, tools abound, but knowledge of them isn't a given.

For me, what works best is a combination of mainstream and alternative/natural medicine. Neither sector has all of the answers. Each is vital in its own way. Like a shield and a helmet fortifying a warrior, they're armor for the woman battling a mood disorder.

Ultimately, I want my experiences to relay hope and encouragement. I pushed back against my illness and found people who listened to me. So can you. Along the way, I discovered a path that led to healing. So can you. At the end of the day, hope and encouragement sustain us as we plow through the minefields of mood disorders.

The same hope and encouragement echo in the stories of the many women I've interviewed. Two of those stories round out the rest of this chapter, and show how different people find different ways to overcome their illnesses and heal.

What Worked for Amy: Conventional Medicine and Psychotherapy

Well before she became a mother, Amy struggled with depression.[23] She first noticed signs of it when she was 7 years old. To manage her symptoms, she took Prozac. Two years before she got pregnant, she slowly weaned off of the medication, because she didn't want it to affect the baby. Given her history, it wasn't a shock when depression surfaced during pregnancy.

In the absence of the medicine, she suffered. She didn't sleep well, she cried nearly every day, and she frequently felt suicidal. Yet, she strived to hide her plight. She did so successfully, until a nurse asked her to fill out a questionnaire on depression. Amy answered the questions truthfully and admitted she was fighting depression. The nurse moved fast to get her into a psychiatric evaluation, and called a firefighter for help. Amy just as quickly enlisted the help of her own psychologist, who explained to the nurse that they'd been working together weekly to manage her depression. This prevented her from being hospitalized. "It was just a terrifying experience. I didn't know that's how it worked. I would have lied on the depression survey if I knew I would be taken by force by a firefighter to the hospital," she says. Her psychologist believed hospitalization would be traumatic and sought to help her avoid it.

Meanwhile, Amy and her husband had their home remodeled during the pregnancy. They lived with her parents until shortly before the baby arrived. The moving around didn't allow her to develop a routine as she entered motherhood, and added another layer of instability to her life.

During childbirth, her daughter swallowed amniotic fluid. The baby went to the neonatal intensive care unit (NICU) for

---

23 Amy's real name has been changed to protect her privacy.

one day, where she was hooked up to tubes that monitored her breathing. Amy was born prematurely herself, and she already was sensitive to complications that might arise. The NICU experience also dashed her hopes of immediate breastfeeding and bonding with the baby.

The first 2 weeks were smooth, when her husband took time off from his job. After he returned to work, she grew afraid to be alone with the baby. Nursing was fraught with problems. The baby didn't latch properly, and although Amy breastfed her regularly, she didn't gain weight. When the baby was 3 weeks old, Amy saw a lactation consultant on a Sunday. "The lactation consultant panicked." Together they called the child's pediatrician, who suggested formula for a day, but the lactation consultant—who argued that the child should go to the ER—won. Amy took her daughter to the ER for tests and analysis. "It was 5 hours of torture," she says. "Deep down, I knew all she needed to do was eat."

As the nursing problems waxed, her sleep waned. Pumping and feeding every 3 hours meant she didn't get more than an hour of slumber at a time. Still, she continued nursing, partly in response to family pressure, and partly due to her own beliefs. She thought using formula would be like poisoning her child, and that it'd be too expensive. "I kept telling everyone it wasn't sustainable. My mom and my husband pressured me to continue with the breast milk," she says. At the end of 4 weeks, she was unable to sleep at all. "I thought I would be a terrible person if I gave my baby formula. I was going to do whatever it took to not give my baby formula, but unfortunately that did me in."

Compounding the mental anguish was an abdominal sprain that had happened during labor, something that wasn't diagnosed until months later. The abdominal pain made it even more difficult to sleep. She says,

> I didn't know if the pain would ever go away, if the
> baby would sleep, if I would sleep. I wasn't getting

better on my own. I was getting worse and worse.
... My family just didn't understand. I kept telling
them it was too hard to not sleep. My husband
suggested staying awake for 24 hours, and I tried
it, and it backfired.

Amy became suicidal and homicidal. She reached what she calls
"ground zero" when she admitted her homicidal feelings to her
mother. Her mother shared the information with her father, who
then told her husband. Although she had previously tried to tell
him she wasn't doing well, he didn't realize the severity of her
suffering. At her parents' urging, Amy called her psychiatrist,
who was often booked one month in advance. Her psychiatrist
did a phone session with her that day, which was a Thursday, and
set up an in-person appointment with her the following Tuesday.
That day on the phone, she didn't discuss the homicidal or suicidal
thoughts with her psychiatrist. If she had done so, she believes the
doctor would've referred her on the spot for an in-patient evaluation, which Amy didn't want. So she only conveyed her lack of
sleep and that she was depressed. The doctor prescribed Prozac,
and she started taking it right away. But she still wasn't able to sleep.

At the in-person session with her psychiatrist, she ultimately
shared her suicidal and homicidal thoughts. Her doctor determined that she needed to go to a psychiatric hospital for an
evaluation: "She called my husband and told him he had to make
an appointment for me that day. She told my husband and my
parents that I could not be left alone with the baby." In addition to
the Prozac, Amy began taking Seroquel, an antipsychotic medication. For the first time in a month, she slept for 8 hours straight.

After the evaluation, Amy's psychiatrist enrolled her in a
partial-hospitalization program: "The kindest option she [the
psychiatrist] could give me was partial hospitalization, and it was
only because she had a good relationship with me." Normally, her

psychiatrist would've suggested inpatient hospitalization. The doctor advised the part-time program primarily because she knew Amy had a strong support system at home, and that either her husband or her parents could be with her at all times.

For 3 weeks, she went to the hospital for treatment during the day, and returned home in the evenings. As part of the program, she participated in group and individual therapy, learning techniques like mindfulness, and focusing on positive thoughts. She also took art therapy and drew pictures that reflected her emotions. She met with a psychiatrist regularly, who adjusted the doses of her medication based on her symptoms. Amy's mother and husband cared for the baby. Because she was on medication, she stopped nursing, one of the hardest choices she's ever made.

At first, she went through the motions of the partial-hospitalization program, hoping eventually she'd feel better. In time, she did. The medication began to work, she regained sleep, and she developed a schedule with routines. She finished the program when her daughter was about eleven weeks old, and she felt well enough to return to her job. "I did really well with the schedule and having time away from taking care of a baby. Having a job was essential for my recovery," she says. Getting back to the things she was used to doing, like her work, brought constancy and relief. She also continued to see her psychologist after the partial program, to continue individual therapy.

She stopped taking Seroquel after a few months, and now uses Klonopin on an as-needed basis, to help her sleep. As of this writing, Amy still takes Prozac, and her depression is in remission. She says her health and family life are in a good place, and she hopes to have a second child.

Looking back, she wishes a few things had been different. For example, she wonders why no one—including the lactation consultant—encouraged her to pump an extra bottle of milk and ask her husband to use it for a night feeding, so she could get extra sleep. She believes such a simple solution would've gone a long way to helping her cope. She now shares that advice with expecting and new mothers.

She also believes she would've been better off if she'd sought help while she was pregnant. Stigma, she says, prevented her from acting: "If I had gotten help then, I probably wouldn't have experienced what I did postpartum. I would have already been on medication, or it wouldn't have happened." The stigma still sticks. Amy asked for her real name to be withheld, because she doesn't want to invite judgment based on one set of circumstances in her life. "I really feel strongly that there is a lot of prejudice toward people with depression, and stigma."

Ultimately, Amy is grateful that she found the help she needed. She believes conventional medicine is the best line of immediate defense when a mental illness is life-threatening. Amy credits psychotherapy with both her short- and longer-term healing. All of her therapy—before she became pregnant, as part of the partial-hospitalization program, and afterward—has made a difference. "Just recently, my husband remarked that I viewed and reacted to life situations in a healthier way," she explains, which he believes might not be the case if she hadn't gone through the partial hospitalization. She says,

> While I do not wish the experience on anyone, it did cause me to address unhealthy thought behaviors in a completely focused way, and I made a decision to change my thoughts from negative thoughts to positive ... more decisively than I had in the past. It has changed the way I live my life.

What Worked for Melissa:
Naturopathic Medicine

Melissa Bangs[24] experienced postpartum psychosis after the birth of her daughter, Adelaide, in 2012. She was 40 at the time of the birth. It was essentially flawless—a gentle, 10-hour birth at home, during which she was joined by her husband, Eric, and their midwife. Melissa didn't need any stitches, something for which she'd been striving. Happily, she eased into a brief-but-cozy pre-storm calm.

The psychosis came on gradually, over the course of a month, and increased as Melissa's sleep debt grew. What started as weepiness continued throughout the month, and was followed by intrusive thoughts and hypervigilance: "I really unreasonably felt it was my job to never let her [the baby] cry." To that end, she would nurture and soothe Adelaide all day, and not put her down. Meanwhile, Melissa neglected her own needs, including eating and drinking water.

Eventually, she "went to this other reality. I would describe it as an experience of pure love. I felt like I could hear and see and feel the vibration and frequency in living and inanimate objects. I felt I was a channel to ancient truths." On a chilly day in October, her midwife came to visit, and found her sitting outside on the ground, wearing only her bathrobe. Adelaide was with her, safely bundled and warm. Although she wasn't experiencing paranoia or dark thoughts, Melissa wasn't functioning at a level where she was adequately taking care of herself or the baby.

Her midwife stayed with her until her husband arrived home from work. He called her parents, who came over, and together they all went to the emergency room. There, Melissa was put on several stabilizing medications. "They said that I needed to go

---

24 My personal communication with Melissa Bangs took place between November 5, 2015, and May 18, 2016.

to the psych ward. So I was put in a van with a couple of large, friendly men who drove me to the psych ward," she says. Her family followed, and she was admitted.

Melissa stayed in the psychiatric hospital for 3 ½ weeks. During that time, she and her family didn't have a say in the treatment she received. She says:

> I am grateful for the safe space I was provided, and the energy and care of the people around me. People were incredibly dedicated to their jobs. They worked really hard. They were kind. I absolutely needed to be stabilized, and I eventually was. But the care was not adequate.

She points to three specific inadequacies in her treatment at the psychiatric hospital. The first relates to her extreme sleep deprivation. Doctors tried Melissa on nine different drugs, from mood stabilizers and psychotropic medications to those that aided with sleep. They sought a formula to stabilize her. Instead, she believes they should've first addressed her lack of sleep by administering only sleep medication for the first few days—something suggested by a recent study on the treatment of postpartum psychosis. (For more on this, see Chapter 5.) Another shortcoming was that the hospital failed to test her hormone levels. Melissa's hormone balance ultimately played a key role in her healing, once she was under the care of a naturopath.

The third issue was limited time with Adelaide. Because the facility didn't specialize in PMADs, there was no special time reserved for mother-baby visits, so Adelaide came during regular visiting hours, which meant 30 to 60 minutes every day or every other day: "During those visits, my psychiatrist would decide if I was allowed to hold her or not." The approach didn't recognize how detrimental that separation can be—on its own—to a new mother's mental health. It wasn't nearly enough, she says, to protect the invaluable mother-baby bond that develops in the early days of a child's life. The separation was the most painful experience of Melissa's life. "The baby was the most vulnerable being I had ever met, and she needed me, not anyone else, and I wasn't there. I was just gone, and we had no power and no say," she says.

In the hospital, her symptoms continued. She heard voices saying a variety of things, among them, "There's no such thing as time and space—these are manmade constructs," and, "Everyone you've ever loved is here, now." She describes ethereal experiences of intuition, where she believed she could see what people around her had lived through in the past. If time was just an illusion, she thought that by re-enacting her daughter's birth, she could travel through time, and wake up to the moment her daughter was born. "I attempted to rebirth Adelaide three times in the psych ward. With the primal scream and everything," she says.

The faithful support of her husband and family were a lifeline. They visited her in the hospital several times a day. Melissa's aunt, who lived out of state and had been a psychiatric nurse, offered her help through phone calls. Although they didn't make decisions on her treatment, she says, her family's constant presence, and their willingness to ask questions and share their informed opinions, created accountability among the hospital staff caring for her.

Her family gave the clinical team a sense of the safe, supportive community to which she would return. Melissa says,

> They were an essential part of the safety plan and the reason the psych team felt very secure in sending me home. Also, they were essential in helping that team identify when I had returned to myself. That team didn't know me, but my family did.

Melissa's biggest source of strength—from the time she fell ill until she was fully well—was her husband Eric. He was at her side the entire way. He was strong and loving enough to take her to the hospital when he was afraid, and he didn't have the tools to help bring her back to herself. He was patient throughout her hospital stay, she says, waiting to see the woman he recognized while "advocating for the woman he loved. If a drug or set of drugs sent me far from myself ... paranoia, fogginess, forgetful, disjointed ... he spoke up, he shared that this wasn't me and wasn't working."

His strength and presence played a fundamental part in her being sent home: "I wouldn't have found my way back to myself without the incredible support, love, and non-judgment of my husband." He never made her feel as if it were her fault, as if she were "somehow damaged or crazy"—this was one of his greatest gifts. She says, "he never had a moment where he let on that he thought I wouldn't be returning healthy, whole, and complete."

At the end of Melissa's time in the hospital, the psychiatrist who treated her diagnosed her as having bipolar disorder. He sent her home on two medications, lithium and Trilafon, a combination her care team believed would keep her stable and help her sleep.

Once she left the hospital, she shared what she learned with her aunt and her aunt's colleague, who was a psychiatrist. After they both reviewed her case, they agreed the bipolar diagnosis was wrong. Instead, they believed she suffered from postpartum psychosis. She later imparted this to another psychiatrist, one she was required to see within 3 days of leaving the hospital. The visit was horrendous. The psychiatrist didn't have time to review Melissa's case beforehand, so she entered the conversation relatively uninformed. When Melissa posited the possibility that she had postpartum psychosis and wasn't bipolar, the psychiatrist dismissed it: "She talked to me as if I were a manipulative 5-year-old child."

Melissa's frustration rests solely with that psychiatrist. She doesn't intend it as commentary on the entire field of psychiatry. While the diagnosis and treatment she received from the psychiatrist in the hospital didn't hold the keys to her ultimate healing, she continues to like and respect him, and she's grateful for his help.

As the lithium took effect, she experienced a time she describes as emotionally "flat," when she was unable to feel love for Adelaide. She also battled anxiety and insomnia—neither of which was prompted by the lithium. When her husband was away on business, different family members would spend the night and help care for the baby.

Determined to feel better and not return to the psychiatric hospital, she sought alternatives. She first consulted with a naturopath who recommended a gentle line of treatment that would take about three years to render her healed—too long. Her midwife then took her to see a different naturopath, Dr. Christine White. "She is the care provider that brought me back to stasis. Without her, I can't imagine what my life would look like," Melissa says.

Dr. White ran a panel of tests, examining and addressing all of her hormone levels and neurotransmitters. The results stunned them both. Her levels of estrogen, progesterone, serotonin, melatonin, and dopamine were extremely low, while her testosterone and adrenaline were quite high, and her cortisol levels spiked every night. Using vitamins, minerals, herbs, nutrients, naturopathic remedies, and bioidentical hormones, Dr. White treated each hormonal imbalance and Melissa's insomnia. Soon, she was sleeping well. Within a few weeks, her anxiety faded to nothing. Two months after she launched into the new line of treatment, she stopped taking lithium.

Melissa and her husband also developed "a safety plan" in case her psychosis flared up again. Elements of the plan included:

- ▸ a therapist with PMAD expertise;
- ▸ a psychiatrist to call if there were a crisis;
- ▸ access to medication;
- ▸ an alternative safe place instead of the psych ward; and

> ▶ an agreement regarding the particular scenarios in which her family would put her back in the psych ward: "This wasn't a La La Land choice made from a place of denial. I simply gave my heart/mind/body the chance to find out if I would be okay without lithium."

Having a say in her treatment made all the difference for Melissa: "Dr. White invited me into a conversation about my care. She educated me and gave me options." The approach was refreshingly different from what she found in the psychiatric hospital. Melissa says a mother must be given the chance to listen to her body and her instincts. Then, along with information and options from skilled health care providers, and the loving support of family and friends, she can make a choice. If that doesn't happen, she's likely to feel powerless, and her body's ability to heal will shut down. Melissa says:

> Postpartum, we are so vulnerable. There has to be room in that path and that vulnerable, tender, bewildering time to be given an opportunity to advocate for our own health and our own journey back to ourselves. While we are extremely vulnerable, we are extremely fierce, and that can't be lost.

Still, at certain points during her illness, Melissa could not have made choices for herself. "I didn't and was not able, and counted on loved ones to educate themselves and advocate for me. Even the decision to put me in the psych ward was an act of love," she says.

Melissa is grateful for the way her story has turned out. She thrives on the time she spends with Adelaide, and she works part-time as a storyteller and an advocate for maternal mental health. She recognizes that her experience could've been more severe. It wasn't until she started sharing her experience that she developed an appreciation for what other psychosis survivors endure. "In the realm of psychoses, I got off really lucky," she says. "I was lucky in that I didn't hurt myself, and I didn't hurt Adelaide." She points to the other grueling layers often part of psychosis, cases where women make repeated trips into and out of psychiatric hospitals, not finding the care they need, years lapsing as they search for answers that'll bring stability. They might be on the wrong medication, or medication that leaves them in emotional shambles, feeling like foreigners in their own bodies and far from the high-functioning, vibrant people they once were.

Out of these ruinous truths, Melissa is building pillars of knowledge, understanding, and hope. The vehicle through which she's doing this is a one-woman storytelling performance, "Playing Monopoly with God," in which she details her journey through postpartum psychosis. Melissa is a masterful story-teller. Her show doesn't just address the sad points—it reveals the surprisingly funny side too, and she winds both into a well-rounded recounting of agony and loss, gratitude and gain. Mostly, she imparts strength, the knowingness of someone who has loved, lost, and come victoriously to the other side of a terrifying experience. Her show reminds us all of the importance of sharing our postpartum stories, no matter how long or large our fears loom. She's performed the show across Montana, and as of this writing, she'll take it on a West Coast tour.

In addition to the show, Melissa conducts storytelling workshops for mothers of all ages who encountered a traumatic or difficult postpartum period. She also collaborates with Dr. White. Together, they hope to improve postpartum care for suffering mothers. They believe women should be better informed when it comes to their treatment options and educated on less-well-known subjects, like hormonal imbalances and what naturopathic medicine offers.

To date, Melissa hasn't had another episode of any kind. She prioritizes sleep, eats well, hydrates, and takes care of herself.

Healing: A Lifelong Endeavor

True healing is a work in progress, as the women in this chapter exemplify. They confronted their illnesses and the emotional fallout left behind. Teresa Twomey, who had postpartum psychosis and wrote a book about it, refers to this as two levels of healing:

> There is the recovery from the psychosis and then there is the recovery from having had this illness— the learning to trust yourself again, dealing with the fear of a recurrence, being tormented by questions of "why me?" and so on. The illness is temporary—women recover from it relatively quickly. However, the emotional pain from having had this illness can last a lifetime (Hale, 2009).

After Teresa wrote her book, she sent psychosis survivors a survey related to their recoveries. The most common response she received was that the women hadn't healed emotionally. Some had psychosis several decades ago, and they were still in pain. Teresa said in an email exchange, "Some even made comments indicating regular and persistent anxiety and/or grief, mourning over the time lost with their child (that is, time they were not emotionally present, not necessarily about physical presence, although some expressed both)" (T. M. Twomey, personal communication, January 29, 2016).

Teresa discusses the stages in the context of postpartum psychosis, but any woman with a PMAD should walk through both stages. Yet, I suspect many do not. Emotional wounds linger and fester well beyond the baby years. They might be written off as hormonal fluctuations or monthly cycles, or as adjustment to the ceaseless challenges of motherhood.

We must do better.

As the stories in this book show, healing is a team effort. When we ask for and receive help from others, it's a process of grace with the power to save: husbands, family, and friends who don't give up on us; caregivers who understand; and others who know that when it comes to mental health, one size doesn't fit all. When our footing suddenly slips, we cling to these grounding social supports. Consider Melissa Bangs, who says the rock-solid foundation she had in her husband and the rest of her family was central to her recovery.

We must be kinder to ourselves.

Healing from any trauma, loss, or pain—including what we experience postpartum—takes a lifetime. It will alter us forever. That doesn't mean emotional affliction will be our permanent plight, or that we won't feel fully well. It does mean that as we strive for our best mental and physical health, we should give ourselves room to grow and change. My own emotional healing and growth continue, not in spite of suffering, but because of it. One of my favorite verses says,

> Not only so, but we also glory in our sufferings, because we know that suffering produces persever-ance; perseverance, character; and character, hope. And hope does not put us to shame, because God's love has been poured out into our hearts through the Holy Spirit, who has been given to us (Romans 5:3-5, New International Version).

Suffering is an intruder that invades our lives and threatens our very existence. But it also comes bearing the unlikely gifts of perseverance, character, and hope. These are gifts we can offer to others, especially hope. When we make known the times we've suffered and what got us through them, we extend hope to those listening. If they're able to tap into that hope when they're facing hardship, if it helps them get through, and they later pass hope to more people—then affliction has immeasurable value.

CHAPTER 9

Getting There

Where We've Been, and Where We Need to Go

Every day you may make progress. Every step may be fruitful. Yet there will stretch out before you an ever-lengthening, ever-ascending, ever-improving path. You know you will never get to the end of the journey. But this, so far from discouraging, only adds to the joy and glory of the climb.

SIR WINSTON CHURCHILL,
Painting as a Pastime

In March 2016, American astronaut Scott Kelly returned to earth after 340 days in space. He detailed his journey by sharing show-stopping photos from his heavenly perch. Among the images on his Twitter feed is one of the Himalayan mountains, captured a few days before the end of his mission. Along with the picture he wrote, "The #himalayas remind me of the bigger view we see when we conquer the #mountains we climb" (Kelly, 2016). Spending almost a year off the planet and living to tell about it is a mountain he climbed and conquered. No doubt, Kelly's travels enriched his life with a broader perspective on many things. His voyage and analogy remind me what it was like to live through the traumatic birth of my first child, and the aftermath. Childbirth jettisoned me into an alien postpartum world, pocked by mental pits and black holes. My familiar life was far from view. Some days I wondered if I'd ever shake the sense that a stranger had invaded my body, if any kind of normalcy would resurface.

Thankfully, the chaos of my mind quieted. Once it did, I had a clearer sense of the delicacy of the human brain. My walk through postpartum depression afforded me time to stop and consider where I had been, and where I wanted to go.

One place I wanted to go involved writing this book. I was determined to better understand PMADs, and uncover resources for women struggling through them. While doing so, I've discovered two central truths. We've made significant strides in terms of awareness and quality of care—but mountains remain for us to climb and conquer.

The people who serve families struggling with PMADs go to great lengths to help them get the care they need to recover, heal, and lead productive lives. Brave, benevolent women and men— Katie Kmiecik, Mark Williams, and Teresa Twomey, to name a few—after fighting their own battles, have devoted their lives to helping others afflicted with mental illness. Education continues to increase about the tools available to new parents, including therapy and prescription medication, support groups, and alternative medicine and therapies.

Progress is evident at the institutional level too. In 2000, the first perinatal partial-hospital program in the United States opened in Rhode Island. More have cropped up since. We now have a total of eight intensive outpatient/partial-hospitalization perinatal psychiatric programs, and three inpatient programs (see the side-bar in this chapter, "Doing More for New Mothers"). Although U.S. inpatient programs don't allow babies to stay overnight, children do spend time with their mothers as part of the treatment, and to promote healthy bonding. Other parts of the world have offered inpatient perinatal programs for quite a bit longer, known as mother-and-baby units, or MBUs. MBUs let infants stay with their mothers around the clock.

All of this good work is encouraging. But we still have much to accomplish. We must improve education for health care providers and the general public, as well as screening and prevention efforts. Changing the way PMADs are discussed, both formally and informally, is crucial. In the United States, increasing the number of psychiatric-care facilities specifically for PMADs would make a world of difference. Underlying all of this is what we do about stigma. No matter how hard we work, I doubt humanity will ever see a day when mental illness is free from stigma's iron-grip. But we can loosen it. The most effective way is by talking. When we share our own stories, and listen to others' stories, we light the way with education, understanding, hope, and healing—all the while driving back the darkness and shame.

Mountains We Have Climbed

Of all the accounts parents have shared, one stands out as a keen example of how a family stricken by a PMAD should be treated. Lindsay MacGregor, a London-based mother and wife, was recovering from severe postnatal depression and postpartum psychosis when I spoke with her and her husband, Alasdair.[25] Lindsay fell ill after the birth of their first child, Leo, in February 2015.

The couple had tried to get pregnant for nearly a year, to no avail. After a string of stressful life events, including the loss of one of Alasdair's brothers, they quit their jobs and set out to travel for a year. Five months into their adventures, Lindsay got pregnant—likely, she says, because she finally relaxed. Though she and Alasdair were surprised by her PMADs, she now believes there were red flags during her pregnancy, but she didn't recognize them as such.

Morning sickness, for instance, kicked in with an unusual bang. Both a psychological and physical illness, it was characterized by a lack of positive outlook, extreme fatigue, disorientation, bleak thoughts, a struggle to carry out basic tasks like washing and eating, and her skin hurt when touched. "It didn't look like morning sickness I'd read about anywhere. It went on from 7 weeks to 18 to 19 weeks, and I was pretty much bedridden. I had not had depression before," Lindsay says.

No issues arose in the second-half of her pregnancy, and the couple returned to London 2 months before she gave birth. As part of the health care offered by the UK's National Health Service (NHS), a team of midwives is assigned to the part of London where they live. One midwife visited them at home once Lindsay was in labor, and said she was dilated by a few centimeters. They found it

---

25 My personal communication with Lindsay and Alasdair MacGregor took place between October 29, 2015, and May 25, 2016.

odd when the midwife instructed her to remain laboring at home. After an exam, a midwife in her specific area of London typically accompanies a laboring mother to the hospital, and will then be her assigned midwife for the birth. Lindsay ended up going to the hospital without her assigned midwife, who went off duty a few hours later.

After laboring at home for 24 hours, the couple made a chaotic journey to the hospital. Lindsay was so far along, she couldn't stand upright. One of Alasdair's brothers came to the couple's aid and drove them in their van to the hospital. Lindsay, meanwhile, crouched on all fours in the back as Alasdair helped keep her steady from the front passenger seat. Once at the hospital, Lindsay took nitrous oxide and sat in a warm bath to mollify the pain. A team of "absolutely wonderful" midwives tended to her, and by then she'd been in labor close to twenty-eight hours. She says,

> In between contractions, we were laughing and having a great time. We bonded with the midwives. They were very special ladies. By the time they asked me to push, I was so exhausted, I couldn't get Leo out, and Leo was getting into a bit of distress.

The baby was delivered with the help of a vacuum extractor. He was healthy and Lindsay was relieved, but exhausted. Her postpartum care in the hospital was "good but short." The couple's student midwife came to visit even after she was done with her shift, and a nurse brought in the placenta so they could see it. "There were so many super people in my experience, super-special people," Lindsay says. "I came home with Leo 48 hours later, and things were fine for a while."

Complications emerged once Lindsay went home. She developed mastitis, accompanied by a fever, and was put on antibiotics to treat the infection. While out for a walk, she had sharp, contraction-like pains, and quickly returned home, where she delivered an errant part of the placenta. Soon, she was taking more antibiotics to ward off another infection. For about ten days, her mother looked after Leo. Meanwhile, Lindsay was growing fatigued and irritable with the baby. She started to smoke—something quite out of character: "Something clicked in my brain, and I felt like I'd turned into somebody else." Over the next several days, she started chain-smoking. She couldn't eat, sleep, or take care of the baby. Then came the convulsions— sudden, violent jerks of her arm hitting her head.

Initially, Lindsay and Alasdair visited their doctor, who prescribed her sertraline, an antidepressant safe for her to use while nursing. But her condition deteriorated. Alasdair recalls that, "On the weekend, the depression and convulsions got worse—she was endlessly smoking and in her bathroom all day. On Sunday, she was lying on the floor, convulsing." Not wanting to wait until Monday morning to return to the doctor's office, Alasdair took her to the accident and emergency (A&E) department of their local hospital (the equivalent of an ER). They were quickly moved into a private room, where they waited for a few hours for the psychiatric doctor to arrive. Alasdair says,

> Lindsay was lying on the floor and groaning, and
> jumping, very strange and intense and primal. She
> had moments of clarity where I could talk to her.
> It was like pulling back a curtain, and then the
> curtain would come down.

In the week leading up to their time in the A&E, all of Lindsay's conversations with Alasdair were circular and paranoid, a cycle he couldn't stop. "There were no words of consolation that could end it. I was always reassuring her—it was like the conversation hadn't happened before," he says. Their conversations in the A&E were the most trying. When the psychiatric doctor arrived—a gentle, lovely man named Tim—he arranged for Lindsay and Leo to be transferred the next day to the Channi Kumar Mother and Baby Unit at the Bethlem Royal Hospital. Reflecting on her ride to the mother-and-baby unit (MBU), Lindsay recalls being in the ambulance, unable to control her movements: "Every single movement hurt me so badly that I couldn't imagine getting through the next moment. It was continuous pain."

A mental-health nurse greeted Lindsay on her arrival at Bethlem, and showed her around: "I describe it as strangely like a boarding school. The rooms are really nice—a kitchen, a lounge and a huge area, a nursery, where we got round-the-clock care for our babies." When she entered the MBU, Lindsay could barely function, and she'd lost all feeling for her son. The medical staff increased her dose of sertraline. They also prescribed a strong antihistamine to help her sleep, and Diazepam to treat her anxiety. "For me, a huge part of my recovery [was] the other women in the unit. They were from all walks of life," Lindsay says. One woman, for instance, was an asylum-seeker from Somalia who'd just had her third child and didn't speak English. Lindsay says:

> We'd be in a room washing the babies, feeding the babies, or watching TV, or sitting and eating not-great-but-free food. We had nothing in common, except that we couldn't pretend in any way to be perfect mothers. I felt a solidarity with those women that I haven't felt with any women in my community since. I felt like I learned how to be a good mother in that unit, around those women and the nurses, who had years of experience and loved Leo when I couldn't love him.

A male nurse who had five grown daughters of his own connected especially well with Leo. "He was an invaluable male presence in Leo's early life. ... He cried when we left, and we cried. He'd bonded so much with Leo," Lindsay remembers. For her, life at the MBU was like living in a village. With every aspect of the baby's care, she was around other women, and she learned from them: "We were sharing resources, and it felt so right. When everything else felt wrong, it felt right—the way they were doing things there. I do miss that camaraderie hugely."

Quite simply, Lindsay says, the 12 weeks she and Leo spent at the MBU saved her life: "I've never asked for help before. But here I asked for help, and in every way, I've been given the help I needed." The MBU was life-altering for Alasdair too. He says,

> For me the place was absolutely crucial. It was explicit support. I didn't have to stress about leaving work, taking weeks off work. I didn't have to get up in the night, so I was sleeping well and resting well and exercising. So I was able to be healthy and happy, which made *me* a better support. I was able to be the best version of myself, so when I would go see her, I wasn't caught up in the whirlwind of her illness—which I would've been if I'd been stuck at home. I was supported, joyful. I loved going [to the MBU] and sitting on the sofa and watching crappy TV and talking to the wonderful babies. Just wonderful characters you make friends with. It was an amazing thing.

Alasdair enjoyed the support of an understanding employer, who didn't balk when he left work a bit early several times a week. This gave him time to get to the MBU, which was across town, by 6 p.m. to be with Lindsay and Leo. He felt very welcome at the unit. "We were to leave at 8 p.m. every night, but not once did anyone ask me to leave. I usually left around 8:20 or so. ... And I think that's really significant, them not asking me to leave." Alasdair also spent most weekends at the MBU.

For Lindsay, her husband was the anchor that steadied her through the storm. "I never felt like he didn't understand," she says. She describes him as "rare among his peers," willing and able to discuss his feelings, and quick to extend empathy. As soon as Lindsay's behavior shifted, he knew something was amiss with her health. He didn't see it as a stain on her character, or as a weakness. "I was worried, but I knew that it wasn't Lindsay. And I knew it was something that was happening to her, and something we would get through and come out stronger on the other side," Alasdair says.

The only glitch in her care, Lindsay says, was with the medicine. "I kept saying every week, 'I think the sertraline is causing me anxiety,' and they upped the dose and they didn't respond. I didn't push it, because I'd never been on antidepressants," she says. After about ten weeks, she grew angry, prompting her doctors to change her medication. They weaned her from the sertraline and tapered in the Effexor, and within a few days, she felt better. She wonders what would've happened if she had taken the Effexor at the outset. "And that's the problem with not knowing," she says. "All of this is new—I didn't know when I should push back. I didn't feel empowered enough to push back in the right areas. Now I push back."

Lindsay returned home after 12 weeks at the MBU, and felt ready to leave. "I think day by day it's getting better. I've had a couple of relapses corresponding with PMS, but generally things are really good. My default setting is pretty positive and pretty joyous."

It's still difficult for her to grasp what she lived through. But she believes even if she'd "had an easy birth and 20 nannies, it would've happened. At some point, my brain just broke and chemically something just went wrong." The experience has made the couple stronger as individuals, and better parents. It allowed Lindsay the freedom to grow into the mother she always wanted to be. She says,

There's a push in modern society for the way you should be as a mother, and it doesn't look anything like the way I am when I'm instinctively mothering. Going into the unit and taking away all of that, and being a real mum and [not caring] what others were saying—I feel very free as a mother now.

Mother-and-Baby Units Abroad

Lindsay's time at the MBU made all the difference in her recovery and healing, and in her family's health and well-being. Her experience isn't the norm, however. Most women don't have access to such facilities, let alone funds to cover the significant costs involved. To understand why, it's helpful to take a closer look at MBUs: their history, where they're located, and how they operate.

The United Kingdom—a leader in perinatal mental health care—is the birthplace of the MBU. According to an article in the *Archives of Women's Mental Health,*

Chronologically, for historical reasons, Great Britain has pioneered in the perinatal area. This began in the very particular setting of England after the Second World War. The evacuation that moved children out of London during the Blitz revealed the harmful effects of separating families. Thereafter it became routine practice to admit mothers and young children together to paediatric hospitals. This practice facilitated the first joint psychiatric admission of a mother and baby, in 1948, for a woman suffering from non-psychotic depression. Gradually, in the years that followed, women with all kinds of mental illnesses related to childbearing were admitted to special units set up in adult psychiatric departments (Cazas & Glangeaud-Freudenthal, 2004, pp. 53-58).

In 1959, the UK's Banstead Hospital opened the first separate MBU: "Psychiatrists there observed that psychotic mothers hospitalised with their children could be discharged sooner and had fewer relapses than psychotic women admitted alone without their infant into an adult psychiatric unit" (Glangeaud-Freudenthal et al., 2014, p. 149). The UK's Maternal Mental Health Alliance lists 17 MBUs, including 15 in England and two in Scotland (n.d.).

A 2009 study of England's MBUs defined them as inpatient psychiatric units that can admit mothers and babies, have at least four beds, and are separate from other wards (Elkin et al.). The units are supported 7 days a week, 24 hours a day by multi-disciplinary staff tending to both mothers and children. Most MBUs in the UK and France are attached to public hospitals—either general or psychiatric. The units can be located in a variety of settings, such as separate buildings, as part of larger units of psychiatry, near maternity wards, or in pediatric units (Glangeaud-Freudenthal et al., 2014).

It was in 1960 that joint full-time admissions first happened in France (Cazas & Glangeaud-Freudenthal, 2004). A child psychiatrist spearheaded the country's first MBU, which opened in Créteil, near Paris, in 1979. More MBUs opened in the years that followed, also promoted by child psychiatrists. France defines an MBU by three criteria:

1. The dual goal of caring for women's psychiatric disorders while also facilitating mother-baby interaction and bonding;

2. Trained, multi-disciplinary staff specific to the unit; and

3. A secure location for the mother and child (Glangeaud-Freudenthal et al., 2014).

Beginning in the early 1980s, public inpatient MBUs developed in Australia, and Belgium's first MBU opened in 1985 (Glangeaud-Freudenthal et al., 2014).

Some countries have only one or two MBUs, typically with five to eight beds, including the Netherlands, Hungary, Sri Lanka, and India. In Luxembourg, Israel, and Switzerland, individual arrangements are established when a mother requires inpatient treatment. They're admitted together with their infant to unspecialized psychiatric wards. In other cases, a single MBU has opened for a few years or less and then closed, as in Canada and New Zealand. Germany offers therapy at inpatient units or day clinics, and if needed, joint mother-baby admissions (Glangeaud-Freudenthal et al., 2014).

Structure, Operations, and Staff

Full-time MBUs typically treat mothers with severe mental illnesses while allowing their children to stay with them. There's beauty and benefit in this:

> Care in an MBU may lessen the effect of maternal problems on the child's development. Remaining with their babies during psychiatric treatment should prevent the potential detrimental effects to the baby of separation from the mother, and the effects this separation could have on the mother's self-confidence. Most women admitted with their babies are pleased that they need not be separated from their child while receiving care in an MBU, a finding that confirms "the central importance women with severe mental illness assign to motherhood" (Glangeaud-Freudenthal et al., 2014, p. 148).

The last point is particularly important for deflecting stigma. Mothers with PMADs are easily castigated. They may be thought of as crazy, self-absorbed women who don't care about their children. But a mother fighting postpartum depression doesn't love her child any less than a mother fighting cancer. Each is an unwanted illness. Neither is an indication of character. We need to remember to share this with others who might not know it.

An MBU must be structured to provide mental health care for mothers in addition to care for infants "that will enable secure child development. The units should also facilitate interaction between parents and infant and enable the father to participate in the child's care and interact with him" (Glangeaud-Freudenthal et al., 2014, p. 151).

The goal isn't always to keep a mother and child together despite risk. It is, however, to provide time, a safe place, and support as they develop or restore a good relationship. Sometimes separation is necessary. Here again, the MBU plays an important role. It gives those involved the gift of time—to find the best placement for the baby, and to help the mother accept it (Glangeaud-Freudenthal et al., 2014).

Caregivers in the units have demanding jobs that require multiple skills, as they look after both adults with mental-health conditions and babies. While a consensus hasn't been reached regarding how to structure and staff the units, those versed in MBUs agree: Staffers need proper training and continuing education to perform their jobs well. The suggested size of an MBU is between five to six beds. This enables the best organization of staff and doesn't overwhelm the patients.

Studies have shown that in France, Belgium, and the UK, between 63 and 78 percent of women demonstrate marked improvement by the time they leave MBUs, despite the different types of care offered between countries. Once women leave, they need continued care to sustain their recoveries and guard against relapses (Glangeaud-Freudenthal et al., 2014).

Although they're separate entities, MBUs don't operate in a vacuum. To achieve things like training and education for staff,

and appropriate follow-up care for patients, they have to collaborate closely with adult and child psychiatric wards, obstetricians,
other maternity-unit staff, and pediatricians. MBUs should be
part of a network of medical and social services. This facilitates
referrals and follow-ups for patients once they're discharged back
into the community (Glangeaud-Freudenthal et al., 2014).

Despite reported success of MBUs, much research remains to
determine best practices and cost-effectiveness:

> The UK model for specialised perinatal mental
> health services emphasise the need for properly
> integrated mother-baby inpatient units and peri-
> natal community psychiatric teams to ensure that
> the needs of mothers and their infants are met
> both before, during, and after inpatient care. At
> the same times, the regional variation in avail-
> ability within individual countries and between
> countries is striking. No evidence-based guidelines
> are available for structure, staff, or practices in
> MBUs, and no assessment of the most effective
> practices for prevention and for mental health care
> of the mother, the baby and their family. Although
> it is a financial and methodological challenge,
> short and long-term evaluation of the cost-effec-
> tiveness of such units is needed compared with
> other treatment options, for women with mental
> illnesses who need inpatient treatment, either in
> a day centre or alone in an adult psychiatric unit,
> with the child cared for elsewhere (Glangeaud-
> Freudenthal et al., 2014, p. 153-154).

Without proof of cost-effectiveness, it's difficult to help policy
makers understand why they should commit to funding MBUs
(Glangeaud-Freudenthal et al., 2014).

A Closer Look: MBUs in the UK

The United Kingdom has been a leader in maternal mental health care, and continues to push for progress. In early 2016, British Prime Minister David Cameron announced that almost a billion pounds would be poured into improving mental-health services nationwide (British Prime Minister's Office). As part of the plan, 290 million pounds is intended for creating new community perinatal mental health teams and additional beds in MBUs (Campbell, 2016).

Dr. Trudi Seneviratne,[26] consultant psychiatrist and lead clinician at the Channi Kumar MBU at Bethlem Royal Hospital, where Lindsay MacGregor was treated, says during the last decade, the perinatal mental health community has diligently raised awareness for its cause. This has influenced the culture, and how much value it places on perinatal mental health. Cameron's announcements indicate the government is finally recognizing the impact of PMADs. When a mother struggles with poor mental health, Seneviratne says it affects "the development of the child, and the child gets psychological problems. So the cost to society is so much more that way around."

Women admitted to Bethlem's MBU have severe illnesses that can't be managed at home, through visits with a nurse or clinic. The illnesses can include anxiety, depression, psychosis, obsessive-compulsive disorder, and emotional instability. When the MBU handles cases of psychosis, the mother most often is confronting it for the first time in her life. Seneviratne says,

> Some people get a very mild version, some get a
> very severe version. It's too risky to ask the family
> to manage it at home because of the rapid deterio-
> ration. The rates [are] 1 to 2 per 1,000 deliveries, but

---

26   My personal communication with Dr. Trudi Seneviratne took place between December 28, 2015, and March 21, 2016.

it's common enough that we see it. The prognosis in recovery is very good.

The cornerstone of care for all women, no matter what their illness, is keeping them with their babies: "It's the separation that can be very traumatic, and recovery takes that much longer. ... It really makes a difference to keep mother and baby there. It makes a difference for both the mother and the child." Separation can have emotionally devastating consequences. She explains:

> [If] mom and baby are separated for 6 months, it's very hard to develop the mother-baby bond. We know from attachment theory the early weeks and months are really important. The beauty of the MBU is that even if the mother is very sick with psychosis, the mom can dip into as much care of the baby as she can do. The nurses will gently encourage her to do as much care as possible, so the baby receives quite a bit of time from the mother throughout the day.

The average length of stay is between 8 and 12 weeks. For the last 5 years, the unit has served between 70 and 90 patients each year. "Our unit is always full. We could do with another one in south London," Seneviratne says. The goal, however, is to build at least another three MBUs in areas of the country where none currently exist. This will help eliminate the need for women to travel long distances for proper care. That's important, Seneviratne says. Although her MBU receives referrals from all over the UK, including Wales and Scotland, and can admit faraway patients in severe circumstances, women often don't want to travel.

With 13 beds, Bethlem houses the country's largest MBU. Though expansion is possible, Seneviratne says it would only be by a few beds. "There's something about the optimal size of the unit. We might be able to stretch it to 15. You can't stretch it beyond that, because the psychology of the work is so intense."

Seneviratne thrives in her role as lead clinician. "I know that's where my strengths are, rather than the research. I'm looking after patients, and after services, and educating," she says. Eight other specialists serve the MBU, including academics and full-time clinicians, and there's a total staff of about 50 caregivers. Although the first line of treatment is medication, the general approach to treatment and recovery is holistic. This includes a variety of alternative therapies, such as art and dance, family/couples' therapy, occupational therapy, baby massage, gentle exercise, and healthy eating. According to Seneviratne,

> When the moms are on the unit is not the time for psychotherapy—it might be something they plug into later on. The sort of women that come into the unit are on the severe end of the spectrum. They might have very severe anxiety or depression, or they might have a psychotic illness or bipolar illness, and they've relapsed and become manic. We have a lot of women who develop psychosis— so they are bipolar, or they develop psychosis with no previous mental-health issues.

These women are agitated, and their thought processes are blocked, so the last thing they want to do is sit and talk. Even patients who talk for a living, such as a university lecturer who developed psychosis, may not want to engage in talk therapy. "This mom didn't want to talk," Seneviratne says. Instead, exercise and alternative therapies were instrumental in her recovery. "We are very lucky, because our unit is very holistic."

The MBU works to bolster the mental health of the entire family. "We really reach out to dads on our unit," she says. "About a third of dads get depressed if their wives have postpartum depression." But men who suffer from depression aren't likely to discuss it. "Perinatal mental health is about the family, not just treating the mom. You are thinking about the baby, the partner. So our focus is to engage the partner as much as possible." PMADs strain marital relationships, and the MBU staff, trained in family therapy, are sensitive to this. They aim to work with couples on issues that arise, and sometimes grandparents are included, as well.

The element of time plays a key role in healing and recovery, a principle on which Seneviratne won't budge. Around ten years ago, there was a push throughout the UK to shorten how long patients spend in MBUs, to 4 or 6 weeks. "I stood my ground and said, 'There's no way I'm going to shorten our length of stay.' Things like anxiety and depression disorder take weeks to lift. We can't turn them around in a couple of weeks," she says.

If a mother is sent home too soon, she leaves lacking confidence and knowledge about how to care for her baby. An 8-to-12-week stay allows the mother to get well, heal, and develop parenting skills and self-confidence. Around week seven or eight, there's a discharge planning meeting to determine how the mother will re-enter life outside the unit. A community psychiatric nurse, a psychiatric doctor, and a children's social worker are assigned to each patient on leaving.

Ideally, Seneviratne says, the time to focus on a woman's mental health isn't after she has a baby—it's from the moment she conceives the child: "Depression is probably just as common in pregnancy. So we want to help midwives detect women depressed in pregnancy and offer treatment then. And we might be able to refine the treatment while [they're] pregnant."

The Bethlem MBU serves a large portion of south London through a perinatal team of caregivers, such as midwives and general practitioners. The team conducts house visits, and identifies women at risk of developing perinatal mood and anxiety disorders. They do so with an eye on reducing the chances that a woman will be stricken with a severe PMAD and need treatment at the unit. If these measures don't stave off an illness entirely, they might at least shrink the severity of the symptoms.

Pioneering Roots

UK Psychiatrist Champions Perinatal Mental Health

It was under the wing of one of the pioneers of perinatal mental health, Dr. Ramesh "Channi" Kumar, that Dr. Trudi Seneviratne launched her work at the Bethlem MBU. She joined him in the late 1990s, to conduct research on postnatal depression. Back in 1981, Kumar had been appointed consultant in charge of the then-new unit (Bugra, 2000). He held that post until he died in 2000, and also was a professor of perinatal psychiatry at the Institute of Psychiatry at King's College London.

An article in the *British Journal of Psychiatry* says,

> Channi was a key figure in the development of perinatal psychiatry as a specialty, and his research into the causes, consequences and treatment of postnatal mental illness gained him an international reputation. One of his greatest achievements was in raising awareness—in public, medical and academic arenas—about postnatal mental illness and its impact not only on the women who suffer from it but also on their babies and other family members (Marks, 2004, p. s1).

Kumar was one of the founders of The Marcé Society for Perinatal Mental Health, an international group, and served as its second president, from 1984 to 1986 (Marks, 2004).

America's Answer to the MBU

The United States lags other countries when it comes to perinatal mental health care. Compared to the UK's 17 inpatient MBUs and France's 20, we have just three, none of which allow babies to stay overnight with their mothers. The length of stay is shorter, too—days instead of months. We do have experts dedicated to providing excellent care for families battling perinatal mood and anxiety disorders, and they've succeeded in their endeavors. We just need more of them.

Leading the Way: Rhode Island's Day Hospital

One such expert is Dr. Margaret Howard,[27] director of the Day Hospital and Women's Behavioral Health at Women and Infants Hospital in Providence, Rhode Island. The Day Hospital, which opened in 2000, was America's first perinatal partial-hospital program for pregnant women and new mothers with depression, anxiety, or other emotional distress. Before the Day Hospital launched, Howard and her colleagues saw a gap in mental health care for new mothers. She says,

> These were women that needed much more inten-
> sive treatment than once-a-week outpatient [care].
> So we would send them to traditional partial-hos-
> pital programs and they would leave after the first
> day, or they wouldn't even go. They were separated
> from their babies, and they were with a mixed
> psychiatric population.

It was evident that they needed more specialized care. The answer came in the form of a perinatal partial-hospital program. "We are fundamentally different from the European MBUs. In European MBUs, moms and babies will stay 12 weeks or beyond, while in our program, it's closer to 12 days."

The Women and Infants Hospital that houses the partial program is a specialty hospital for women and newborns. The

---

27   My personal communication with Dr. Margaret Howard took place between February 23, 2016, and May 23, 2016.

eleventh-largest stand-alone obstetrical service in the United States, it sees nearly 8,400 deliveries each year—more than 70 percent of all of the births in Rhode Island, according to Howard: "There aren't a lot of other maternity wards in the state. We have an excellent reputation as an academic teaching hospital. Yet it has a community-hospital feel." Back when the Day Hospital was taking shape, hospital leadership embraced the idea, which took 3 years to develop, a time of extensive planning and study. She says:

> We did the best we could in creating a program we thought would meet the needs of the women. We had no other model but the European model. I was confident in our clinical team and that they would provide high-quality, expert care. I had no doubts whatsoever about the care these women would get. Before we opened, we had to convince all the major health insurers that this was a highly needed and worthwhile venture, and imperative that it be covered service.

Being closely aligned with the OB/GYN community at Women and Infants has been key to the program's success—most referrals originate from obstetrical providers and word-of-mouth. Women are identified during OB visits, after they have a baby, or when they self-identify. Others come from private psychiatric hospitals, private practitioners, and pediatricians, and some from out of state. Howard says,

> Coming to Women and Infants for your perinatal mental health treatment is more palatable to a lot of women than going to a traditional psychiatric setting. Because PPD is widely regarded as the most common complication of childbearing, I am a real champion of the notion that mental-health treatment [should be] part of the continuum

of obstetrical care, albeit provided by perinatal mental health specialists.

A partial-hospital program, such as that offered by the Day Hospital, is just one step down from an inpatient unit, Howard says, the only difference being that patients go home to sleep. Mothers come in with their babies every weekday, Monday through Friday, and spend up to 6 hours each day. Howard is an avid supporter of the model. By sending the woman home to her family at night, her caregivers can gauge her progress and whether the treatment is effective. For example, a mother evaluated on the first day may say she's so depressed she hasn't read a book to her toddler in 6 weeks, she hasn't showered in a week, or she spends inordinate amounts of time yelling at her partner. By day 4 of her treatment, if she says she's reading to her toddler, showering, sleeping in larger increments, and is no longer as quarrelsome—these are clear signs that the treatment is taking hold.

Another upside is cost. "In this country, partial hospitalization is far less costly than inpatient hospitalization. The aim of the Affordable Care Act is to reduce costs, while ensuring high-quality care and high patient satisfaction, which we believe our model accomplishes," according to Howard.

All of the women who come to the Day Hospital battle some form of a perinatal mood and/or anxiety disorder. They often struggle with mother-baby attachment, so the program focuses intently on helping them establish a secure, healthy bond with their infants or soon-to-be-born infants. "These moms suffer. They feel enormous guilt," Howard says. Clinicians carefully evaluate each referral to recommend appropriate treatment, setting, and plan of care. If the recommendation and agreed-on plan mean a patient is admitted to the Day Hospital, she'll pursue an intense treatment plan tailored to her needs, including individual therapy, medication management, and skill building. The program also offers family therapy, consultation on nutrition and lactation, and personalized outpatient care plans for discharge. If necessary, program staff make referrals for colic, and other infant-health and mental-health issues. "Women get better fairly quickly, and that's our goal: to stabilize them," Howard says.

On average, a patient's length of stay is around ten to fourteen days. To determine when a patient is ready to move on, the program uses concrete benchmarks that coincide with her presenting problems and treatment plan: "We look for improvement in mood, overall functioning, future-orientation, and a lessening or absence of her presenting symptoms." Family meetings are especially helpful, because they offer additional insights and observations on how a patient's treatment is progressing.

As to the program's success, numbers tell the story. In 2014, the Day Hospital moved into a larger space and added staff, which has allowed it to double the number of patients it hosts each day: 13, on average. The expansion was a longtime coming, Howard says. The facility had reached its maximum capacity after 4 or 5 years of operating, and women who needed treatment were placed on a waiting list.

U.S. perinatal mental health programs should be more widely available than they currently are, Howard says: "At the very least, there should be one in every state. Women, no matter where they live, should have access." She believes Europe is far more advanced on this front than America. One thing stalling us is stigma. When a topic snags the public eye, through awareness campaigns and dedicated treatment facilities, for instance, "everyone starts talking about it. That's when the stigma goes down. France and the UK have had MBUs dating back generations. People know about them, and [PMADs get] de-stigmatized," Howard says. "There's far less stigma in Europe, and also in

Australia, and this may be due to the widespread availability and longevity of specialized treatment programs."

Howard has made some remarkable discoveries since the Day Hospital took flight:

> What I've been most struck with is the healing power of mothers coming together at a time in their lives when society expects them to be so happy, and yet they are suffering tremendously. They're depressed, unhappy, anxious, and not functioning, and basically feeling miserable at a time the world is telling them they should feel great. These women experience a profound sense of isolation and inadequacy. And to come together and be with other women who are feeling the same thing, to recognize that they are not alone is so, so powerful. It's not what we professionals with our fancy degrees have to say to them. It's what they say to each other.

If a woman faces a perinatal mood disorder, it doesn't mean she's a bad mother, that she's defective, or didn't want her child—these truths bear repeating. Howard says:

> The other thing I've learned in a very big way is that these conditions are very treatable, and that women get better. As a professional working in this field, it is enormously rewarding to see women get better. It's huge. And they're grateful, too. Some women can't fathom feeling anything other than suffering. To see them come out of that is rewarding. A lot of what we do early on is instill hope ... and let them know they're not alone.

Breaking New Ground: UNC's Inpatient Unit

Perinatal inpatient psychiatry programs in the United States are few and far between. To date, we have programs in North Carolina, California, and New York (see the side-bar in this chapter, "Doing More for New Mothers"). North Carolina's facility was the first to open, in 2011. Serving mothers with the most severe PMADs, it's a free-standing unit at the University of North Carolina at Chapel Hill.

Getting an inpatient program off the ground is no easy feat. It must be financially viable and sustainable, and ensure the patients' safety. Proving all of this to insurance companies is essential. While Europe's MBUs make a strong case for admitting both the mother and child, it's a complicated question in the United States, a fundamentally different place than other countries. Dr. Wendy Davis, executive director of Postpartum Support International, says, "I believe the main reason that we are not more advanced in having MBUs with babies is related to how litigious our country is." Liability insurance for U.S. medical providers and hospitals is extremely expensive. According to Davis,

> The concern always voiced by a hospital is, "What's our liability? How much will it cost to be insured for the safety of infants in a hospital setting, when we're treating a woman who needs treatment for (mental health)?" So it's about the liability and cost of liability insurance.

That babies aren't allowed overnight at U.S. inpatient facilities doesn't indicate that the babies aren't wanted. Quite the contrary, Davis says. She believes staffing hospitals would relish the chance to set up European-style MBUs, were it not for liability and the cost of insurance.

Christena Raines,[28] perinatal psychiatric nurse practitioner and assistant professor at UNC's perinatal psychiatry program, agrees with Davis: Liability and financial issues prevent the UNC facility from admitting infants. She says,

> From a financial standpoint, we can't do it like Europe. There's no insurance company here in the States that would [cover] a 3-month stay. And from a liability standpoint, we'd have to have specialized staff just to take care of the baby. We feel it's important to include the baby, but not be the primary caregiver. That's what happens in the European units. They provide a lot of care for the babies.

As to whether babies will be allowed overnight in the future—a common question—Raines doesn't foresee such a day, given how cost-prohibitive it is. Still, the program understands and supports the need for a mother and child to be together, and it provides for that as much as possible: "What we do offer is flexible visiting hours." If a mother wakes up at 2 a.m. and wants to see or nurse her child, one of her adult family members can bring the baby to her. A family house is connected to the hospital, where patients' relatives can stay with the baby, at a reduced rate. This is especially helpful for out-of-state families, placing them in close proximity.

For the UNC program to morph from concept to reality required the convergence of several factors, not the least of which was experts who backed the effort. "Pulling together the people in a system [who are] willing to work hard and be passionate and continue to push is the most important part," Raines says. The leading champion who started the program is Dr. Samantha Meltzer-Brody, director of the perinatal psychiatry program at

---

28   My personal communication with Christena Raines took place between February 27, 2016, and October 17, 2016.

UNC's Center for Women's Mood Disorders. Her research on MBUs in Europe and Australia informed the process. Meanwhile, Raines says, UNC staff made a discovery. When their perinatal patients were treated in general psychiatric units they were stabilized, but a gap remained. Because the treatment wasn't specific to PMADs, the women felt they weren't getting an education to help them understand what was happening to them. Although they have some similar components, PMADs and generalized depression are quite different. "Moms want to know why they have this. So we wanted a more comprehensive unit for the perinatal patient," Raines says. A pilot program showed that an inpatient facility could be viable and sustainable:

> [W]e decided we'd develop 2 weeks' worth of programming to address the needs specifically of the perinatal patient. They'd get the psychological education they need to understand the disease process, to understand why things are happening—as much as we know why things are happening—and equip them with the skills they need once they are discharged. Our goal was not to have them fully healed, but well on their way to recovery, with the tools they need to continue and heal.

Protecting patients' sleep was a driver in the decision to go with the inpatient format. "We needed an inpatient [unit] where patients could stay overnight, and feel safe and have the ability to rest, because sleep is one of the important medicines we can [give] these moms," Raines says.

The UNC program receives referrals from all over the country for its five beds, and there's a waiting list. In 2015, it treated between 100 to 120 patients. What often holds patients back is insurance not willing to pay for treatment out of their home states.

Mental health care providers refer patients, who are assessed by UNC staff.

Once a patient is admitted to the program, a team of highly trained doctors, nurses, psychologists, midwives, social workers, and other therapists collaborate to develop an individualized treatment plan for her. Treatment includes medication management, supportive therapy, education for a patient and her family, occupational therapy, spirituality and nutritional counseling, and recreational therapy, such as yoga, relaxation, and biofeedback. A critical point of treatment is sleep. "Sleep is a type of medicine—it is the number-one medicine," Raines says. Adequate sleep can help reduce the amount of medication a patient takes, and diminish intrusive thoughts. The program wants patients to get at least 4 to 6 hours of sleep at a time. To make sure of that, staff do not measure patients' vital signs every few hours, and treatment plans guarantee a full schedule: "They stay pretty busy. There's not a lot of downtime, and we want that so they can get a good night of sleep."

Timing is critical in treatment, Raines says, pointing to a patient who—despite working in the health field—didn't seek treatment until she was 16 months postpartum:

> It took me a year to get her stable because she had waited so long to get help, out of fear. It's our own judgment and stigma we have inside of our heads that stops us. She just had her second baby, and she's doing great. The longer you wait, the harder it is to treat. With each pregnancy, it gets worse if it's not treated.

Another patient who battled severe depression and intrusive thoughts spent 3 weeks at the unit. She went on to become a doula and a childbirth educator, and developed a module on postpartum depression. The module has helped broach a difficult topic with mothers and families. Too often, educators don't speak of PMADs because they're afraid of scaring new parents. "It's not about scaring anyone. It's about informing people. You don't *not* tell them about postpartum hemorrhage because you don't want to scare them. You tell them," Raines says. Perinatal mood and anxiety disorders are no different from physical maladies, like gestational diabetes or hypertension, and they deserve the same attention. "To me, that is my prime objective—normalizing postpartum depression and seeing it as a complication: treatable, time-limited, and nothing to be afraid of."

The average length of stay is between 7 and 10 days. Program staff strive to make sure each patient has adequate care once she's discharged. After care generally involves a psychiatrist and an outpatient therapist, and it varies based on where the mother lives. If she's native to North Carolina, she returns to the UNC outpatient program. Postpartum Support International helps with out-of-state women, making sure they get appointments with appropriate care providers in their local areas. While UNC does some follow-up, they're working to develop a more comprehensive plan to ensure patients continue on a healing trajectory.

To improve postpartum care for women and reduce stigma, Raines is working on a research initiative called the 4th Trimester Project. The project's website says,

> In the 12 weeks following delivery, a woman must recover from childbirth, adapt to changing hormones, and learn to feed and care for her newborn. During this "4th Trimester," many women experience considerable challenges, including fatigue, pain, breastfeeding difficulties, depression, lack of sexual desire and incontinence. Amid these concerns, postpartum care is often fragmented among maternal and pediatric providers, and 20 to 40% of women do not attend a postpartum visit.

> ... Our goal is to bring together mothers, health
> care providers, and other stakeholders to define
> what families need most during the 4th Trimester
> (University of North Carolina, n.d.).

A goal of the project, according to Raines, is to explore a way of letting all new parents know—regardless of their socioeconomic status—postpartum help is available. That help wouldn't necessarily be in the form of a therapist or a psychiatrist. "Just a mother's friend, or something to tap into that is for everybody, so they don't feel stigmatized reaching out and asking for help," Raines says, pointing out that all people need to be able to call on someone with whom they're comfortable talking. "So many women are falling through the cracks because they don't have the energy, stamina, or understanding to reach out, and the fear is there."

Raines's work at the UNC inpatient unit has shown her how important it is for mothers struggling with PMADs to relate specifically with other women in similar situations. Through their conversations and interactions, mothers in the unit support each other, normalize the feelings associated with mood disorders, and help one another heal. "Facilitating that with these moms has been really important," Raines says. "Being able to talk freely without judgment, and having other moms to talk to ... that's what the unit does for them."

Doing More for New Mothers

Perinatal Psychiatric Programs in the United States

As of this writing, the United States boasts nine intensive outpatient and partial-hospitalization perinatal psychiatric programs, and three inpatient programs. Below is a list of definitions of the different types of programs, according to CARF International

(2016), an independent, nonprofit accreditor of health and human services. Beneath the definitions is a list of the U.S. perinatal programs.

Outpatient treatment programs provide individual, group, and family counseling, and education on wellness, recovery, and resiliency. Intensity of the comprehensive, coordinated, and defined services may vary.

Intensive Outpatient Programs (IOPs) can include treatment during evenings and on weekends and/or interventions delivered by different service providers within a community. An IOP can function as a step-down program from partial hospitalization, detoxification/withdrawal support, or residential services, and it might be used to prevent or minimize the need for more-intense treatment. IOPs are more rigorous than traditional outpatient services.

Partial-hospitalization programs are time-limited and medically supervised, and they offer comprehensive, therapeutically intensive, coordinated, and structured clinical services. They're available at least 5 days a week, but they might also offer half-day, weekend, or evening hours. Treatment includes a series of structured, face-to-face therapeutic sessions at different levels of intensity and frequency. These programs serve as an alternative to inpatient care, as transitional care after an inpatient stay in lieu of continued hospitalization, as a step-down service, or when the severity of symptoms requires such care.

Inpatient treatment programs are 24 hours a day, 7 days a week, with the patient staying onsite in a free-standing or hospital setting. They provide interdisciplinary, coordinated, integrated, medically supervised services. The goal is a protective environment with medical stabilization, support, treatment for psychiatric and/or addictive disorders, supervision, wellness, and transition to ongoing services.

Intensive Outpatient and Partial-Hospitalization Programs

- ▶ Rhode Island's Day Hospital at the Women and Infants Hospital in Providence

- ▶ California's Maternal Outreach Mood Services (MOMS) Program at El Camino Hospital in Mountain View

- ▶ Michigan's Pine Rest Mother and Baby Partial Program in Grand Rapids

- ▶ Minnesota's Hennepin County Medical Center Mother-Baby Program in Minneapolis

- ▶ California's University of California, San Diego Maternal Mental Health Program

- ▶ California's Huntington Hospital Maternal Wellness Program in Pasadena

- ▶ Illinois' AMITA Health Perinatal IOP at Alexian Brothers Women and Children's Hospital in Hoffman Estates

- ▶ New York's Zucker Hillside Hospital, Northwell Health Outpatient Perinatal Psychiatry Services in Glen Oaks

- ▶ New York's South Oaks Hospital, Northwell Health Outpatient and Partial-Hospitalization Perinatal Psychiatry Services in Amityville

Inpatient Programs

- ▶ North Carolina's Perinatal Psychiatry Inpatient Unit at UNC at Chapel Hill

- ▶ California's Perinatal Mood and Anxiety Disorders Program at the Community Hospital Long Beach

- ▶ New York's Zucker Hillside Hospital, Northwell Health Perinatal Psychiatry Services in Glen Oaks

Mountains to Conquer

Recent history has witnessed solid progress in perinatal mental health care. We're no longer stuck in the veritable Dark Ages, a time when we dismissed mentally ill mothers as untouchable and relegated them to the fringes of society. But we've not yet reached a renaissance. Getting there will require hard work, and I'm convinced we can do it.

A good place to start is with our vocabulary, and how we address PMADs, formally and informally. Altering the formal discussion in the American Psychiatric Association's *Diagnostic and Statistical Manual of Mental Disorders (DSM)*, a guiding force in the mental-health world, would be a step in the right direction. The *DSM* doesn't recognize postpartum depression with a unique diagnostic category. It is instead classified under major depressive disorder and through a specifier. A specifier is extra information about a primary diagnosis, which can help caregivers tailor treatment.

Just getting that recognition took time. The 1st edition of the *DSM* was published in 1952. It evolved through several editions, with the latest being the 5th edition (*DSM-5*) in 2013. It wasn't until the *DSM-IV* was published in 1994 that postpartum depression was referred to as "Major Depressive Disorder, with postpartum onset," and postpartum onset was defined as within 4 weeks of delivering a baby, as indicated in an article by Drs. Lisa S. Segre and Wendy Davis (2013, pp. 3-4). The *DSM-5* changed the specifier to "with peripartum onset." Segre and Davis explain the significance of the revision:

> [With peripartum onset] is defined as the most recent episode occurring *during pregnancy* as well as in the four weeks following delivery. This official recognition of depression during pregnancy represents a significant step forward! It is however disappointing that the period following delivery

was not extended to recognize that real suffering
often occurs during the first year, as PSI and others
had lobbied (2013, pp. 5-6).

Davis remains hopeful the time of onset could be changed in
the next edition of the *DSM*. "They considered extending the
4-week onset to 6 months, and they ultimately decided they just
[wouldn't] do it this time. That to me is one thing we really could
push on," Davis says. A mother's symptoms may just begin to arise
at 4 weeks, and peak around three months. "That's something I
really wish they would look at again." One way to make it happen
is by gathering and presenting more research to the committees
of experts who write the *DSM*. This would promote a greater
understanding of how vulnerable women are around the time
of childbirth. "The more research we have about real prevalence
and onset, the better we'll be able to communicate with the *DSM*,"
Davis says.

Other experts agree, and some say the *DSM*'s categorizing of
PPD under the umbrella of major depressive disorder is inaccurate.
Dr. Dana Gossett, chief of the division of obstetrics and gynecology at Northwestern University's Feinberg School of Medicine,
has conducted research on postpartum OCD (for more on this,
see Chapter 4). She says,

> One of the most important things we're learning is
> that women postpartum don't have run-of-the-mill
> depression. It's not the same to have postpartum
> depression as major depressive disorder, because
> there's a lot of anxiety and OCD symptomology. So
> postpartum depression is a lot dirtier. It doesn't fit
> cleanly into *DSM-5* categories.

Gossett says her research has shown this to be true. She's also
concerned by the time of onset listed in the *DSM*:

> We do see mood affects up to a year postpartum. So that seems a really conservative, inadequate definition, because that will miss a huge number of people. When we looked at the people at 6 months [postpartum], some of them had symptoms, but they hadn't had symptoms at 2 weeks [postpartum].

Regardless of the *DSM*, Gossett says it's the less-formal acknowledgment—the social recognition—of PMADs that's fundamental to change:

> I think it's always going to be hard, because at a time when a woman should be joyful, people will always say, "What's the matter with you?" ... Those people aren't reading the *DSM-5*. ... So the social piece—the recognition of this as a real thing, the improved support, that comes more from public awareness than necessarily from the medical community.

In our more informal discussions, it's common to whisk any and all PMADs under the umbrella phrase, "postpartum depression." This can be misleading. To someone unfamiliar with the illnesses, the phrase easily conjures images of a woman who sinks into inexplicable sadness after she has a baby. But there's far more to them. They can arise during pregnancy, not just after childbirth. Then there's the anxiety component. Some say perinatal anxiety is rarely recognized and not often discussed (Rhodes, 2015). By saying "postpartum depression," we gloss over both the timing and the variety of symptoms, and increase the chances for confusion. We should use more encompassing terms, such as "perinatal mood and anxiety disorders" or "perinatal mood disorders." This will shape how we talk and think about PMADs, and ultimately promote greater understanding.

Prevention, Education, and Family Care

We must improve prevention and education. One tool we should use more is screening. In early 2016, the United States saw an important stride toward more comprehensive screening. The U.S. Preventive Services Task Force released recommendations that say pregnant women and new mothers require increased attention in terms of screening for depression (Silberner, 2016; U.S. Preventive Services Task Force, 2016). An NPR article says that the announcement was "part of the panel's recommendation that all adults should be screened, in a situation where they can be provided treatment or get a referral if they are clinically depressed" (Silberner, 2016). Similar recommendations were made in 2002 and 2009. What was different this time was the nod to pregnant women and new mothers. "They need special recognition, the task force says, because of evidence showing that they can be accurately diagnosed and successfully treated, and because untreated depression harms not only the mother, but her child as well" (Silberner, 2016). The panel's move allows for coverage of the screenings under the Affordable Care Act (U.S. Congresswoman Katherine Clark, 2016).

Davis is encouraged by the recommendations. They're pivotal because they indicate perinatal screening "is beneficial to improve outcomes, and there are enough systems and resources in place for us to recommend it." She believes efforts of groups like PSI went a long way to informing the panel's decision. The panel didn't act sooner partly because it wanted assurance that patients in need would get treatment and care. Davis says,

> So now they have seen improved outcomes, risk of harm is minimal, and there are systems in place in the U.S. to handle it. That's our work. It's so encouraging and validating. It helps U.S. providers to say, "We need to consider screening during pregnancy and postpartum because it's that common, and there are places to send them." And now because

of our health-insurance laws, health insurance
cannot bill a patient for that screening.

Screening tools provide a language for both providers and patients
to discuss what's happening, and that reduces the stigma. "That
has been a big shift on the part of medical practice. They were
afraid of making people feel bad by bringing it up," Davis says. But
with more education, the medical world has learned it should be
more concerned about what patients might face if they *don't* raise
the topic of mental health and screening.

Rep. Katherine M. Clark of Massachusetts, who introduced
federal legislation in 2015 for improved screening and treatment
for perinatal depression, called the task force's recommendations
"a major turning point" in how America cares for its families.
"Pregnant women and new moms need to know that they are
not alone, that their suffering matters, and that postpartum
depression can be treated" (U.S. Congresswoman Katherine
Clark, 2016). A senior staffer in Clark's office says the bill has
strong bipartisan support.

These are advances we need. They can help us be proactive,
addressing PMADs before they become severe, and maybe even
before they show up. But as Seneviratne of the UK's Bethlem
MBU pointed out, it's important to track a woman's mental health
from the moment she gets pregnant. Knowing her mental-health
history is key in these screenings too. A woman with previous
mental-health issues needs to let her health care providers know
while she's pregnant, and they should keep this in mind as they
monitor her health. Waiting until the baby arrives can allow a
mood disorder to get a foothold and lead to a world of unneces-
sary hurt.

As with anything in life, knowledge is power, and that's true
for perinatal mental health. By educating health care providers
and new and expecting parents, we can push back against the

illnesses, and give our children a chance to live in a more enlightened world.

Parents need to be educated before the baby arrives. If you're a parent yourself, if you've gone through a PMAD, or your partner did, tell your expecting friends what you learned. Here are the life-changing truths I wish someone had shared with me during my first pregnancy:

▸ **Perinatal mood and anxiety disorders are more common than we realize.** Though the incidence of postpartum depression varies, for instance, based on the population studied and how depression is defined, the typical range is between 12 and 25 percent of new mothers. Some high-risk groups see rates as high as 40 percent or more (Kendall-Tackett, 2016). I mention these statistics not to increase your stress or worry, but as a point of information and awareness. The more you know, the better equipped you can be to advocate for your health.

▸ **If you find yourself wading through a mood disorder, you're in good company.** Plenty of women have had similar experiences. Other moms can be your greatest source of strength. If you have persistent symptoms you know aren't right—intrusive thoughts, sleeplessness, or crying spells, to name some—reach out to a mom you trust. Confide in her. If you don't feel comfortable doing that, contact Postpartum Support International. They have an invaluable network of women who are a phone call away. There's no judgment, shame, or stigma involved.

▸ **A mood disorder is an illness with symptoms, like intrusive images.** The symptoms are treatable, and so is the larger illness, through a variety of interventions like therapy, medication, and alternative treatments.

Physical illness means the body is sick; mental illness means the mind is sick. Psychiatrist and chair of the UK's Maternal Mental Health Alliance, Dr. Alain Gregoire, says it well:

> The reality is that we are all vulnerable to mental illness. Our brains are the most complex structures in the universe and our minds are the uniquely individual products of that structure. It is not surprising then that occasionally things go wrong. The reasons things go wrong are much the same as in physical illness. There may be internal problems such as genetics (we probably all carry some genes for mental illness), infection or the effects of ageing. Most commonly damage comes from the outside (Gregoire, 2016).

▶ **Don't mistake your illness as an indication of your character. Just** because you're not feeling well doesn't mean you're not meant to be a mother, or that subconsciously, you don't want your child. Mood disorders are cunning. They lie. Do not believe them.

▶ **Speak up.** Mental illnesses typically don't go away by themselves—they get worse. Treatment is key, and you shouldn't wait to seek help. Remember, *you* are in charge of your treatment plan. Therapy and medication are the standard line of intervention, but it varies by person. You might not need medication. If you opt to take medicine but it makes you feel worse or has no impact, tell your care providers. When it comes to therapy, consider the different kinds available, including supportive, CBT, and EMDR.

Ask your care providers which would be best for you. If you want to explore alternative therapies, do so—and, as Davis says, be sure you inform your primary caregiver.

▸ **Cling to hope.** Perinatal mood disorders make something that's already difficult—transition to motherhood—more challenging. But they don't last forever. They are temporary and treatable. Ask for help until you find the care you need. Now more than ever, there's an army of people on your side to help you fight back and get better.

Health care providers need more education too, especially those in close touch with new-and-expecting mothers, like OB/GYNs and pediatricians. They should be informed about screening, and how best to support women and their families. Karen Kleiman, founder of The Postpartum Stress Center in Pennsylvania, wrote a piece in *Psychology Today* that serves as a primer on PMADs for health care providers. Kleiman writes,

[M]isinformation permeates our healthcare system like the fog of depression itself. You cannot always see it, but its impact is undeniable, and those who are in the best position to recognize it are not always able to see it for what it is. ... When women are let down by a medical response too misinformed or too preoccupied to take notice, they settle into their fatigue and absorb the incongruity by way of their fragile self-esteem. It must be me. I am flawed. I am not a good mother. It seems so clear to those of us who see these women after being dismissed, condescended to, or misunderstood by their healthcare provider (2015).

To prevent women from slipping through the cracks, Kleiman urges providers to:

▸ Know how common PMADs are, and that they're serious illnesses;

▸ Screen for mood disorders, and work with and refer patients to a qualified specialist;

▸ Understand that postpartum depression is not the baby blues—nor is it postpartum psychosis, but every woman with PPD is at risk for suicide; and

▸ Hold themselves accountable, and equip a patient with reliable resources: "If she is in your office, she is your responsibility" (2015).

Education for the entire family, particularly for a new mother's spouse/partner, is also valuable. Dr. Leslie Butterfield,[29] a clinical psychologist based in Seattle, says we may overlook the impact a mother's mental illness can have on the entire family, including partners, parents, and in-laws. According to Butterfield,

> Women can't heal in a vacuum. They can't get all the healing they need from support groups and from therapy, because the things they go through every day are things in their home. If they can't manage with their partners, if their partners are short-tempered or ill-at-ease, or inside deeply scared about what's going on and feel they can't talk about it—the marriage takes a big hit, and the structure of the family takes a hit.

The U.S. mental health care system, she fears, isn't developed enough to provide adequate care for and inclusion of partners, who often aren't privy to a mother's treatment plan: "She has to go home and tell the partner about her medication and care, because the partner wasn't in the session to hear about the

---

29   My personal communication with Dr. Leslie Butterfield took place between November 3, 2015, and December 18, 2015.

treatment and care." A spouse or partner needs to know, for example, how to care for and support a wife or a girlfriend suffering from perinatal OCD Butterfield says,

> [A]s opposed to getting drawn into the OCD pattern, where the woman is anxious and worried about a lot of things, and then the partner changes how he does things to keep her anxiety down. Which works great for 10 minutes or a day, but which makes the OCD more entrenched than ever. So that kind of treatment needs to be done with family in place—family is part of the treatment team.

Stigma: Just Say No

Stigma is the biggest hurdle we must overcome to improve perinatal mental health care—and care for everyone with mental illness. Even if we don't intend it to, stigma rushes in when we say the words "mental illness." Anyone suffering from an illness of the mind is therefore saddled with disgrace. No wonder so many elect not to share their stories. Languishing in silence seems a lighter load than the burden of shame.

But mental illness is not a disgrace. Not acknowledging this, not doing everything in our power to improve mental health care—that's a disgrace. We can reverse stigma's wrongful tide through big initiatives, such as federal legislation and recommendations. Such sweeping reforms take time, though. In the meantime, change must happen at the individual level, person by person. We can educate one another through discussions on PMADs. We can extend empathy whenever possible. We must honor that having a baby doesn't bring immediate joy to everyone.

Heidi Stevens,[30] lifestyles writer for the *Chicago Tribune*, relayed

---

30   My personal communication with Heidi Stevens took place between September 3, 2015, and September 8, 2015.

her story in one of her columns. She covered important aspects of
perinatal mental health and parenthood in general, and I sought
her out for a phone interview. Stevens says she likely had a mild
case of postpartum depression after her daughter was born. But
she didn't know it until later:

> What I felt was an absence of joy, or comfort, or
> contentment about any of it. I felt like the whole
> thing was sad and hard. I didn't expect that. And
> whether I wasn't educating myself well enough
> on that, or listening to the experts who would
> warn you that it's a possibility, or whether there
> aren't enough experts [warning] that it's a possibil-
> ity—I'm not sure. I felt like I became more tuned
> into the darker, more difficult side of parenting
> after I became a parent.

She believes the inclination to associate happiness with parenthood is wrongheaded. She says,

> I'm sort of done with studies about whether parent-
> ing makes you happy. It's not an emotion you need
> to attach to parenting. It doesn't grasp the whole
> experience. It makes you [feel] many emotions,
> because it's a relationship to a human.

When it comes to the range of emotions related to parenthood, we
need to give each other more space. We tend to be uncomfortable
around grief and unhappiness. Stevens says,

> I have a good friend whose little girl died when
> she was a few months old. She has three kids now.
> People tell her all the time, "You know, you should
> be grateful for what you have." It's a way of saying,
> "Stop dwelling on the sad thing." I think we say
> that a lot, especially about parenting. ... It is a gift
> to get to be somebody's mom. But we shouldn't

tell people they can't acknowledge the hard parts. That's not to say you don't appreciate the gift you've been given.

Stevens believes mental illness carries a lot of stigma in U.S. culture. People often discount the need for medical intervention, she says, and that's especially true with perinatal mental health. For some, it's puzzling that an illness can be triggered by an event—childbirth—that supposedly spells happiness: "It's like, 'What are you talking about, you feel depressed? You got the thing you wanted.'" High-profile cases of mental illness or suicide, such as Robin Williams, set off a temporary buzz. "And then we go back to not really talking much about it."

Having a baby and becoming a mother—these things are dynamic. When we write them off as seasons of life that are simply "happy," we undermine their complexity. Having a baby is painful, grotesque, and every bit as beautiful. Motherhood is difficult, intense, exhausting, and every bit as lovely. It elevates our understanding of life and love in ways nothing else can. When a new mother or father encounters mental illness, it adds to the complexity of the season. It makes life trickier. But human beings are resilient. We heal. The brave women and men in this book prove that. If stigma didn't exist, I wonder how much faster each person afflicted with a PMAD would speak up, get help, and rebound. I pray we reach a day when stigma is reduced to the point where almost everyone understands that an illness of the mind isn't shameful. That would be a true renaissance, where the norm would find new parents getting the help they need quickly, moving on toward healing, and focusing on the bustling business of parenthood.

CHAPTER 10

Better for It

When Postpartum Pain
Is Used for Good

The sad things that happened long ago will always remain part of who we are just as the glad and gracious things will too, but instead of being a burden of guilt, recrimination, and regret that make us constantly stumble as we go, even the saddest things can become, once we have made peace with them, a source of wisdom and strength for the journey that still lies ahead.

FREDERICK BUECHNER, *Telling Secrets*

Just after I lost my brother to severe depression, I read *A Grace Disguised: How the Soul Grows Through Loss* by Jerry Sittser. Sittser, whose wife, daughter, and mother perished in a tragic car accident, discusses his journey through the tragedy, how he coped with its lasting sting, and how he has made sense of his losses over time. At the book's end, he reflects:

> The accident remains now, as it always has been, a horrible experience that did great damage to us and to so many others. It was and will remain a very bad chapter. But the whole of my life is becoming what appears to be a very good book (Sittser, 2004, p. 212).

While Sittser writes about coping with the loss of people, his perspective holds meaning for those of us who have walked through mood disorders, too. Mood disorders lead to different forms of loss—but loss nonetheless. They might cause a temporary loss of self-worth and identity, or a loss of hopes and dreams about how new parenthood will play out. Most importantly, mood disorders rob us of time. I still wish I could reclaim the first weeks of my son's life. If I had another chance, I would do things differently. I wouldn't induce 3 days ahead of his due date. I wouldn't cry my way through his early infancy. I would be more in charge of the situation. Or would I? Hindsight renders perfect vision. If I could travel back in time to who I was on the eve of motherhood, I probably would have followed the same path. So I forgive myself for not being stronger way back then, and forgiveness isn't a singular, said-and-done act. It's a choice I must make, day after day, in my heart and mind.

I'm better for my walk through postpartum depression, and I'm using what I learned to help others. Still, when I look at pictures of me holding a newborn Noah, sweet thoughts of him are like a cordial laced with the bitters of how sad I felt. The veil of time hasn't masked the darkness of those days. The good that continues to develop as a result of my illness doesn't have the power to erase an inherently bad part of my life. Sittser has similar sentiments:

> The accident itself bewilders me as much today as it did three years ago. Much good has come from it, but all the good in the world will never make the accident itself good. It remains a horrible, tragic, and evil event to me (2004, p. 198).

Sittser goes on to say that whatever good comes out of the tragedy, it would never be an adequate explanation or justification that somehow turns the loss into something right or good.

> I do not believe that I lost three members of my family *in order that* I might change for the better, raise three healthy children, or write a book. I still want them back, and I always will, no matter what happens as a result of their deaths (Sittser, 2004, p. 199).

What the experience has shown him is that sorrow and joy, pain and pleasure, death and life—things he once thought of as mutually exclusive—are parts of a greater whole. He writes, "My soul has been stretched. Above all, I have become aware of the power of God's grace and my need for it" (Sittser, 2004, p. 199).

Like Sittser, my closest encounters with grace have been during my darkest days. Grace is mysterious, with a power that leaves me perplexed. Though I have received grace, I struggle to define it. For clarity, I turn to the person I consider the authority: Philip Yancey. He has written books on grace, pain, suffering, and others related to the Christian life. In a Q&A on his website, Yancey offers the best description of grace I have seen:

> As I like to say, grace is a free gift from God, but to receive a gift you must have open hands. You must

sense your own need. ... Unless we face into our own failings and weakness and desperation, we may never receive that gift of grace (2009).

Postpartum depression turned me inside out, revealing my weakness and desperation. I needed something beyond myself to get through it, and I opened my hands for help. Then came grace, furnishing love, support, and care from my family and friends, my OB, and my therapist. I also developed an appreciation for suffering. At some point, in some way—mental, physical, spiritual—we all suffer. As uncomfortable as it is, and as much as we would rather avoid it, suffering has great value. Professor and church historian Kate Bowler said in a 2016 piece in *Christianity Today*, "Suffering that causes you to notice the suffering of others. There's peace in that" (Lee). Bowler, a young wife and mother, knows what it means to suffer. She is critically ill with cancer. She says,

> The weirdest part about being sick is it feels like I can see the secret of the kingdom now. In suffering, you feel God's presence so intensely that you can see how God is trying to draw close at all times. In that sense, it's just an oddly intimate way to experience the suffering of the world, because it's not just yours. You see the brokenness of everything. Before, I was caught up in the sense of my own progress. Now I don't have so many ambitions and desires—because I can't have them. And in that kind of stillness everybody else's pains and hopes become much more real (Lee, 2016).

Three times I have known mental and spiritual suffering: When my mother passed away, when I battled postpartum depression, and when my brother ended his life. With my mother and my brother, I was something of an onlooker. Although their tragic ends significantly altered the landscape of my life, I could only see their pain, not feel it as my own.

My postpartum experience was different. The delicacy of the human mind, how easily breakable we are, how flawed I am, how others endure suffering and pain—these were magnified, and swelled as sad pangs in my heart. No longer just concepts to consider or discuss, they were things I could *feel*. Before, I knew pain, suffering, and brokenness existed, but I preferred to keep them at a distance.

My postpartum upheaval slowed me down and left me no choice but to absorb these things as vital parts of me, coexisting—as Sittser says—with joy, pleasure, and life. Postpartum depression provided a link missing until then: my own acute suffering. At my lowest, I craved stories of lament. They softened the ache in my soul and diminished my sense of loneliness. The Bible's Psalms were life rafts that helped me ride out the waves on a wayward sea of emotions. When I lost my mother and my brother, I was helpless. But not after I had Noah. My actions made a difference. They helped me heal.

It's All About Our Response

Postpartum depression wasn't part of my birth plan. If all had gone as I had anticipated, I would have stayed happily in my comfort zone. That would have meant finding a nanny to help with Noah, and returning to full-time journalism, covering education and business. Writing about perinatal mood disorders wouldn't have occurred to me. My struggle turned mental health into something as precious and personal as my family. I moved forward, knowing that mental health can be a spine-shivering topic. It involves uncomfortable questions that yield unsatisfying answers. Yet, my commitment to the subject enabled me to move beyond my comfort zone, and write about it. There—beyond the edge of where we think we would like to stay—is where we can do life-changing work. It's there that I have crossed paths with remarkable men and women. Some of their stories are in these pages; many others aren't. Connecting with all of them has been a gift. I hope they have found it as healing as I have. This goes back to something Sittser shares near the start of his book:

> It is not, therefore, the *experience* of loss that becomes the defining moment of our lives, for that is as inevitable as death, which is the last loss awaiting us all. It is how we *respond* to loss that matters. That response will largely determine the quality, the direction, and the impact of our lives (Sittser, 2004, p. 17).

As I pushed through postpartum depression, I wanted to find deeper meaning. At first, that meant conversations with other parents and initial research. I soon found that PMADs were more prevalent in and disruptive to people's lives than I had imagined. Many women were afraid to talk. They struggled as a result, often for a long time. It occurred to me that I could help future parents. I could relay my experience, tell them what got me through it, and then do the stuff journalists do: deep research, interviews with other parents, and conversations with experts, tapping their vast reservoirs of knowledge. I would tie it all together into a book that points to the one thing we all need: hope.

My response to loss, then, is this book. It reflects the heart of what I found when I went looking for deeper meaning. God is in the business of recycling bad things into good. He equips us to help in that endeavor. For me, that equipping comes in the form of words. So I write. It's the most effective means I have for extending the comfort I have often received. In the Bible, the Apostle Paul wrote to the Corinthian church:

> Praise be to the God and Father of our Lord Jesus Christ, the Father of compassion and the God of all comfort, who comforts us in all our troubles, so

that we can comfort those in any trouble with the comfort we ourselves receive from God. For just as we share abundantly in the sufferings of Christ, so also our comfort abounds through Christ (2 Corinthians 1:3-5, New International Version).

Whatever your faith, age, or country of origin, whatever perinatal mood disorder you—or someone you love—have battled, I pray that the lasting message you take away from this book is three-fold: comfort, hope, and encouragement. Comfort to remind you that others have passed through similarly ominous depths, and they have survived. Hope to remind you that you too will push through the hardest days and find healing, and ultimately, encouragement to share your story. First, relay it to someone who can help you get well—a trusted family member, a friend, or a clinical caregiver. Second, offer it to other parents who need help, as a way of extending comfort.

As long as women give birth, perinatal mood disorders will trouble us. But they shouldn't have the power to define us, not even for a minute. When I was a young girl fretting over something that no doubt seemed like a trifle to my mother, her remedy was consistent: "Don't worry. Pray." For the postpartum parent worried

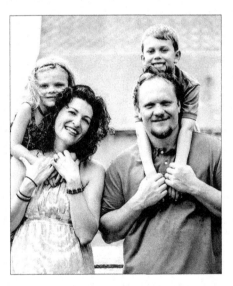

My family: Noah is now 8, and Syma will soon be in kindergarten. Photo by Elisabeth Oda.

at the hands of a mood disorder, I offer this: Don't worry. Pray—*and share your story*. Because it's only in sharing our stories, one by one, that we'll find lasting comfort and true healing.

Resources

What follows is a guide to sources of help for those affected by perinatal mood and anxiety disorders. It is by no means exhaustive. But it does reflect the people and places I believe are on the cutting edge of caring for the afflicted.

Books

The books are organized in two sections. First is a collection of works specifically on perinatal mood and anxiety disorders. After that, you'll find my favorite titles on grief, loss, and the Christian faith.

Books on PMADS

A Deeper Shade of Blue: A Woman's Guide to Recognizing and Treating Depression in Her Childbearing Years, Dr. Ruta Nonacs (367 pages, Simon & Schuster, 2007, paperback, $23.99). A women's mental-health expert explains prenatal and postpartum depression, treatments and self-help, and how friends and family can be supportive.

*

A Mother's Climb Out of Darkness: A Story About Overcoming Postpartum Psychosis, Jennifer Hentz Moyer (263 pages, Praeclarus Press, 2014, paperback, $18.95). Moyer's rich memoir details her experience with postpartum psychosis, and her recovery. It is at once a source of hope, encouragement, and direction for families facing similar battles.

Back in Six Weeks, Sharon Gerdes (294 pages, SKG Press, 2014, paperback, $13.99). This is a novel about a successful career woman who battles postpartum psychosis after the birth of her second child. The author herself had psychosis and is now a mental-health advocate.

*

The Postpartum Husband: Practical Solutions for Living with Postpartum Depression, Karen R. Kleiman (149 pages, Xlibris, 2000, paperback, $20.99). Help and hope for men, from an expert on perinatal mood and anxiety disorders.

*

This Is How We Grow: A Psychologist's Memoir of Loss, Motherhood, and Discovering Self-Worth and Joy, One Season at a Time, Dr. Christina G. Hibbert (430 pages, Oracle Folio Books, 2013, paperback, $19.74). This book covers the life struggles of a clinical psychologist and expert on women's mental health, who also experienced postpartum depression. It illustrates how challenges like PPD can be opportunities for growth.

*

This Isn't What I Expected: Overcoming Postpartum Depression, 2nd edition, Karen R. Kleiman and Dr. Valerie Davis Raskin (317 pages, Da Capo Press, 2013, paperback, $17.99). Postpartum experts share strategies to help women monitor their illnesses, determine when to seek professional help, and find ways to cope and recover.

Understanding Postpartum Psychosis: A Temporary Madness,
Teresa M. Twomey, with Dr. Shoshana Bennett (173 pages,
Praeger, 2009, hardcover, $64). An authoritative account
of what happens during postpartum psychosis, and why.
Twomey, a survivor of psychosis, offers psychological,
personal, medical, legal, and historical perspectives on a
severe form of mental illness that's both preventable and
treatable.

Books on Grief, Loss, and the Christian Faith

A Grace Disguised: How the Soul Grows Through Loss, expanded
edition, Jerry Sittser (237 pages, Zondervan, 2004, hardcover, $19.99). Sittser writes about the bewildering tragedy
that robbed him of his wife, his child, and his mother.
His writing shows how losses as staggering as his don't
have to define us. The crux lies, instead, in our responses
to such losses.

✳

Disappointment with God: Three Questions No One Asks Aloud,
25th anniversary edition, Philip Yancey (336 pages,
Zondervan, 2015, paperback, $6.99). Is God unfair? Is he
silent? Is he hidden? Yancey wrestles with these questions
and assures readers they're not alone in their wondering.

✳

Motherless Daughters: The Legacy of Loss, 20th anniversary edition,
Hope Edelman (400 pages, Da Capo Press, 2014, paperback,
$16.99). Losing a mother changes a woman forever, no matter
how old she is. This book, which helps readers make sense of
the loss and weave it into the fabric of their lives, is an enduring companion.

Motherless Mothers: How Losing a Mother Shapes the Parent You Become, Hope Edelman (448 pages, Harper, 2007, paperback, $15.99). Guidance and support for women who mother children in the absence of their own maternal frame of reference.

✽

Walking on Water: Reflections on Faith and Art, Madeleine L'Engle (256 pages, WaterBrook, 2001, hardcover, $18.99). L'Engle offers a fresh take on what it means to be an artist who follows Christ.

✽

What's So Amazing About Grace? Philip Yancey (304 pages, Zondervan, 2011, paperback, $16.99). Grace is hard to define, despite how often the word is used. An authority on the topic, Yancey takes a humble, brilliant approach that gives readers a firmer grasp on grace, in heart and mind.

Film

Dark Side of the Full Moon, documentary, Maureen Fura, writer/director, and Jennifer Silliman, producer, http://www.darksideofthefullmoon.com/home-1-1

The film examines the state of maternal mental health in the United States, and gives a voice to the untold numbers of women who have silently suffered through PMADs.

Organizations

Healthy Mothers, Healthy Babies Coalition of Palm Beach County

http://www.hmhbpbc.org/

This Florida-based group improves birth outcomes by providing access to prenatal care for uninsured or underinsured pregnant women and teenagers.

✳

National Action Alliance for Suicide Prevention

http://actionallianceforsuicideprevention.org/

This public-private partnership is working to advance a national strategy for suicide prevention.

✳

National Alliance on Mental Illness (NAMI)

http://www.nami.org

NAMI is the country's largest grassroots mental-health organization that strives to help millions of Americans affected by mental illness.

✳

Postpartum Depression Alliance of Illinois

http://www.ppdil.org/

This group promotes awareness, prevention, and treatment of maternal mental health issues. It runs workshops for pregnant women and new mothers, and provides email and phone support to women across Illinois.

Postpartum Progress

http://postpartumprogress.org

Katherine Stone, founder and CEO

This national nonprofit supports women with perinatal mood and anxiety disorders, raises awareness about the illnesses, and reduces stigma associated with them.

✱

Postpartum Support International (PSI)

http://www.postpartum.net

Dr. Wendy Davis, executive director

PSI is a nonprofit organization that promotes awareness, prevention, and treatment of mental-health issues related to childbearing. If you're new to PMADs and looking for help, reach out to PSI first.

✱

The Office on Women's Health (OWH)

http://www.womenshealth.gov

The OWH is part of the U.S. Department of Health and Human Services, and works to improve the health and well-being of all U.S. women and girls.

✱

2020 Mom

http://www.2020mom.org/

2020 Mom is vigorously working to solve the often-unseen maternal mental health crisis affecting many expecting and new mothers. To accomplish that, it strives to influence policy and systems-change by building partnerships, pursuing advocacy opportunities, providing training and tools, and promoting recommendations for hospitals, insurers, and providers.

✱

Prevention and Treatment of Traumatic Childbirth (PATTCh)

http://www.pattch.org

PATTCh is an organization founded by Penny Simkin to disseminate information about birth trauma.

Blogs and Websites

Dr. Will Courtenay, "The Men's Doc"

http://themensdoc.com/

Courtenay is a psychotherapist who specializes in mental health for men and boys. His website touts a variety of useful information, including guidance on paternal postnatal depression.

✱

My Postpartum Voice: Speaking Up, Reaching Out, Inspiring Hope

http://www.mypostpartumvoice.com

Lauren Hale's blog about perinatal mood and anxiety disorders, inspired by her own journey.

✱

Postpartum Progress

http://www.postpartumprogress.com

Katherine Stone's brainchild, and the world's most widely read blog on maternal mental illness. It offers in-depth information, support, and hope for all who have mental illnesses related to pregnancy and childbirth.

Pregnancy and Postpartum Support Minnesota

http://www.ppsupportmn.org/

This is a group of perinatal mental health and psychiatric practitioners who provide support, advocacy, awareness, and training on perinatal mental health in Minnesota. Their website offers community resources and a free peer-support helpline for anyone in need of support or resources.

✻

The Center for Postpartum Health

http://www.postpartumhealth.com

Dr. Diana Barnes, a psychotherapist, started the California-based center to address the psychological and emotional needs of the postpartum woman and her family. She sees individuals, couples, and families.

✻

The Postpartum Stress Center

http://postpartumstress.com

Karen Kleiman founded the Pennsylvania center, which provides support and treatment for the pregnant or postpartum woman and her family, and guidance for her treating physician or therapist.

✻

The Psychologist, the Mom, and Me

http://www.drchristinahibbert.com

The blog of Dr. Christina Hibbert, an Arizona-based clinical psychologist and expert on maternal mental health, grief, and loss. She offers practical, professional guidance, and solace.

International Resources

Dads Matter UK

http://www.dadsmatteruk.org/

A UK-based charity that supports fathers with depression, anxiety, and post-traumatic stress disorder.

✱

Everyone's Business

http://everyonesbusiness.org.uk/

This is a Maternal Mental Health Alliance campaign, calling for all UK women with perinatal mental health problems to get the care they and their families need, wherever and whenever they need it.

✱

Reaching Out

http://www.reachingoutpmh.co.uk/

The website of Mark Williams, a Wales-based mental-health advocate who specializes in helping fathers.

✱

The Marcé Society for Perinatal Mental Health

https://marcesociety.com/

The Marcé Society supports research into and assistance for prenatal and postpartum mental health for mothers, fathers, and their babies.

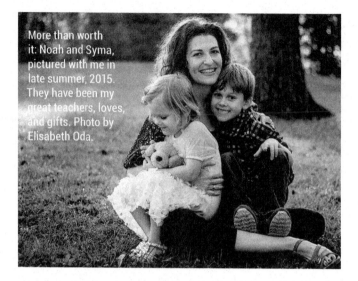

More than worth it: Noah and Syma, pictured with me in late summer, 2015. They have been my great teachers, loves, and gifts. Photo by Elisabeth Oda.

About the Author

Kristina Cowan has been a journalist for 20 years. In the early days, she covered education and policy, first in Chicago and later in Washington, D.C. She was happily back in Chicago by the time she had her first child in 2009. She'd been planning on a baby, but not a traumatic birth or the bout of postpartum depression that followed. It was then that she developed an interest in writing about mental health. It remains at the heart of what she does.

When Postpartum Packs a Punch: Fighting Back and Finding Joy is her first book. She has also written for *The Huffington Post*, AOL, Yahoo, PayScale, Harvard University, the Kellogg School of Management, the American Council on Education, and *Today's Christian Woman*.

She lives in the Chicago area with her husband and two young children.

References

Abramowitz, J. S. (n.d.). *Beyond the blues: Postpartum OCD*. Retrieved from http://beyondocd.org/expert-perspectives/articles/beyond-the-blues-postpartum-ocd

Abramowitz, J. S., Khandker, M., Nelson, C. A., Deacon, B. J., & Rygwall, R. (2006). The role of cognitive factors in the pathogenesis of obsessive–compulsive symptoms: A prospective study. *Behaviour Research and Therapy, 44*(9), 1361–1374. doi:10.1016/j.brat.2005.09.011

Abramowitz, J. S., Taylor, S., & McKay, D. (2009). Obsessive-compulsive disorder. *Lancet, 374*(9688), 491–499. doi:10.1016/S0140-6736(09)60240-3

American College of Obstetricians and Gynecologists and *the American Psychiatric Association*. (2009). *Depression during pregnancy: Treatment recommendations* [News release]. Retrieved from https://www.acog.org/About_ACOG/News_Room/News_Releases/2009/Depression_During_Pregnancy

American Psychiatric Association. (2013). *Diagnostic and statistical manual of mental disorders* (5th ed.). Washington, DC: Author.

Association for Psychological Science. (2013). *Stress hormone foreshadows postpartum depression in new mothers* [News release]. Retrieved from http://www.psychologicalscience.org/index.php/news/releases/stress-hormone-foreshadows-postpartum-depression-in-new-mothers.html

Beck, C. T. (2004). Birth trauma: In the eye of the beholder. *Nursing Research, 53*(1), 28-35. doi:10.1097/00006199-200401000-00005

Beck, C. T., Gable, R. K., Sakala, C., & Declercq, E. R. (2011). Posttraumatic stress disorder in new mothers: Results from a two-stage U.S. national survey. *Birth: Issues in Perinatal Care, 38*(3), 216–227. doi:10.1111/j.1523-536X.2011.00475.x

Belluck, P. (2014, June 16). After baby, an unraveling: A case study in maternal mental illness. *The New York Times*. Retrieved from http://www.nytimes.com/2014/06/17/health/maternal-mental-illness-can-arrive-months-after-baby.html?_r=0

Bergink, V., Burgerhout, K. M., Koorengevel, K. M., Kamperman, A. M., Hoogendijk, W. J., Lambregtse-van den Berg, M. P., & Kushner, S. A. (2015). Treatment of psychosis and mania in the postpartum period. *American Journal of Psychiatry, 172*(2), 115-123. doi:10.1176/appi. ajp.2014.13121652

Bressert, S. (2016). *Delusional disorder symptoms.* Retrieved from http://psychcentral.com/disorders/delusional-disorder-symptoms/

British Prime Minister's Office. (2016). *Prime Minister pledges a revolution in mental health treatment* [Press release]. Retrieved from https://www.gov.uk/government/news/ prime-minister-pledges-a-revolution-in-mental-health-treatment

Bugra, D. (2000, September 19). Ramesh Kumar. *The Guardian.* Retrieved from http://www.theguardian.com/news/2000/sep/20/ guardianobituaries

Bullard, D. (2014). *Bessel van der Kolk on trauma, development and healing.* Retrieved from https://www.psychotherapy.net/interview/ bessel-van-der-kolk-trauma

Campbell, D. (2016, January 10). NHS to give specialist help to tackle mental strain of childbirth. *The Guardian.* Retrieved from http://www.theguardian.com/society/2016/jan/11/ david-cameron-revolution-maternal-mental-health

CARF International. (2016). *2016 behavioral health program descriptions.* Retrieved from http://www.carf.org/Programs/BH/

Cazas, O., & Glangeaud-Freudenthal, N. M.-C. (2004). The history of mother-baby units (MBUs) in France and Belgium and of the French version of the Marcé checklist. *Archives of Women's Mental Health, 7*(1), 53-58. doi:10.1007/s00737-003-0046-0

Darity, Jr., W. A. (Ed.). (2008). Serotonin. *International encyclopedia of the social sciences* (2nd ed., vol. 7). Detroit, MI: Macmillan Reference.

Davé, S., Petersen, I., Sherr, L., & Nazareth, I. (2010). Incidence of maternal and paternal depression in primary care: A cohort study using a primary care database. *Archives of Pediatric & Adolescent Medicine, 164*(11), 1038-1044. doi:10.1001/archpediatrics.2010.184

Denton, J. (2013, October 19). *The absence of light* [Blog post]. Retrieved from https://insideoutjill.wordpress.com/2013/10/19/the-absence-of-light/

Edelman, H. (1994). *Motherless daughters: The legacy of loss.* Reading, MA: Addison-Wesley.

Edelman, H. (2007). *Motherless mothers: How losing a mother shapes the parent you become* (1st paperback ed.). New York: Harper.

Elkin, A., Gilburt, H., Slade, M., Lloyd-Evans, B., Gregoire, A., Johnson, S., & Howard, L. M. (2009). A national survey of psychiatric mother and baby units in England. *Psychiatric Services, 60*(5), 629-633. doi:10.1176/ps.2009.60.5.629

EMDR Institute, Inc. (n.d.). *What is EMDR?* Retrieved from http://www.emdr.com/what-is-emdr/

Frey, R. J. (2012). Serotonin. *Gale encyclopedia of mental health* (3rd ed., vol. 2). Detroit, MI: Gale.

Glangeaud-Freudenthal, N. M.-C., Howard, L. M., & Sutter-Dallay, A.-L. (2014). Treatment – mother–infant inpatient units. *Best Practice & Research Clinical Obstetrics & Gynaecology, 28*(1), 147–157. doi:10.1016/j.bpobgyn.2013.08.015

Gregoire, A. (2016, February 16). These brave mothers' stories must chip away at the stigma of postnatal mental illness. *The Guardian.* Retrieved from http://www.theguardian.com/commentisfree/2016/feb/16/mothers-postnatal-depression-share-story-end-stigma

Grekin, R., & O'Hara, M. W. (2014). Prevalence and risk factors of postpartum posttraumatic stress disorder: A meta-analysis. *Clinical Psychology Review, 34*(5), 389–401. doi:10.1016/j.cpr.2014.05.003

Hahn-Holbrook, J., Dunkel Schetter, C., Arora, C., & Hobel, C. J. (2013). Placental corticotropin-releasing hormone mediates the association between prenatal social support and postpartum depression. *Clinical Psychological Science, 1(3),* 253-265. doi:10.1177/2167702612470646

Hale, L. (2009, April 2). *Sharing the journey with Teresa Twomey* [Blog post]. Retrieved from http://www.mypostpartumvoice.com/2009/04/02/sharing-the-journey-with-teresa-twomey/

Hartocollis, A., & Ruderman, W. (2013, March 14). Mother called her final act 'evil.' *The New York Times.* Retrieved from http://www.nytimes.com/2013/03/15/nyregion/son-survives-cynthia-wachenheims-suicide-jump-in-harlem.html?_r=0

Hawthorne, N. (2011). *The scarlet letter.* New York: HarperCollins.

Hibbert, C. (2014, March 15). *Beyond depression: Diagnosing postpartum OCD–part 2* (and video) [Blog post]. Retrieved from http://www.drchristinahibbert.com/beyond-depression-diagnosing-postpartum-ocd-part-2-video/

Hibbert, C. (n.d.). *Postpartum depression treatment: Sleep.* Retrieved from http://www.drchristinahibbert.com/postpartum-depression-treatment/ppd-sleep/

Hibbert, C. (2012, May 29). *The baby blues and you* [Blog post]. Retrieved from http://www.drchristinahibbert.com/the-baby-blues-and-you

International College of Applied Kinesiology-USA. (n.d.). *What is AK?* Retrieved from http://www.icakusa.com/what-is-ak

Jenike, M. (n.d.). *Medications for OCD.* Retrieved from https://iocdf.org/about-ocd/treatment/meds/

Kahn, M., Fridenson, S., Lerer, R., Bar-Haim, Y., & Sadeh, A. (2014). Effects of one night of induced night-wakings versus sleep restriction on sustained attention and mood: a pilot study. *Sleep Medicine, 15*(7), 825–832. doi:10.1016/j.sleep.2014.03.016

Kelly, S. (2016, February 24). *The #himalayas remind me of the bigger view we see when we conquer the #mountains we climb. #YearInSpace.* Retrieved from https://twitter.com/stationcdrkelly/status/702565434495782914

Kendall-Tackett, K. A. (2016). *Depression in new mothers: Causes, consequences and treatment alternatives* (3rd ed.). Abingdon, UK and New York: Routledge.

Kleiman, K. R. (2015, June 30). *Postpartum depression: Whose problem is it?* [Blog post]. Retrieved from https://www.psychologytoday.com/blog/isnt-what-i-expected/201506/postpartum-depression-whose-problem-is-it

Kleiman, K. R., & Raskin, V. D. (2013). *This isn't what I expected: Overcoming postpartum depression* (2nd ed.). Boston, MA: Da Capo Press.

Lanza di Scalea, T., & Wisner, K. L. (2009). Antidepressant medication use during breastfeeding. *Clinical Obstetrics and Gynecology, 52*(3), 483-497. doi:10.1097/GRF.0b013e3181b52bd6

Lat, D. (2013, March 15). *In defense of the suicidal Columbia Law mother* [Blog post]. Retrieved from http://abovethelaw.com/2013/03/in-defense-of-the-suicidal-columbia-law-mother

Lee, M. (2016, February 23). On dying and reckoning with the prosperity gospel. *Christianity Today.* Retrieved from http://www.christianitytoday.com/ct/2016/february-web-only/kate-bowler-on-dying-and-sure-hope.html

Lemay, G. (2009, August 20). *The undervalued therapeutic power of rest* [Blog post]. Retrieved from http://wisewomanwayofbirth.com/the-undervalued-therapeutic-power-of-rest/

L'Engle, M. (2001). *Walking on water: Reflections on faith and art.* Colorado Springs, CO: WaterBrook.

Lindahl, V., Pearson, J. L., & Colpe, L. (2005). Prevalence of suicidality during pregnancy and the postpartum. *Archives of Women's Mental Health, 8*(2), 77-87. doi:10.1007/s00737-005-0080-1

Marks, M. N. (2004). Introduction: Professor Channi Kumar (1938-2000). *British Journal of Psychiatry, 184*(46), s1-s2. doi:10.1192/bjp.184.46.s1

Maternal Mental Health Alliance. (n.d.). *Mother and baby units.* Retrieved from http://everyonesbusiness.org.uk/?page_id=349

Mayo Clinic. (2015, April 8). *Slide show: Vaginal tears in childbirth.* Retrieved from http://www.mayoclinic.org/healthy-lifestyle/labor-and-delivery/multimedia/vaginal-tears/sls-20077129

Mayo Clinic Staff. (2015, August 11). *Postpartum depression: Complications.* Retrieved from http://www.mayoclinic.org/diseases-conditions/postpartum-depression/basics/complications/con-20029130

Mayo Clinic Staff. (2015, July 3). *Vacuum extraction.* Retrieved from http://www.mayoclinic.org/tests-procedures/vacuum-extraction/basics/definition/prc-20020448

Miller, E. S., Chu, C., Gollan, J., & Gossett, D. R. (2013). Obsessive-compulsive symptoms during the postpartum period: A prospective cohort. *Journal of Reproductive Medicine, 58*(3-4), 115-122. pmid: 23539879

Moreland, J., & Coombs, J. (2000). Promoting and supporting breast-feeding. *American Family Physician, 61*(7), 2093-2100. Retrieved from http://www.aafp.org/afp/2000/0401/p2093.html#afp20000401p2093-b30

National Health Service. (n.d.). *Health visitor.* Retrieved from https://www.healthcareers.nhs.uk/explore-roles/public-health/health-visitor

National Library of Medicine. (2014, July 28). *Placenta previa.* Retrieved from https://medlineplus.gov/ency/article/000900.htm

National Library of Medicine. (2014, November 15). *Sertraline.* Retrieved from https://medlineplus.gov/druginfo/meds/a697048.html

Neufeldt, V., & Guralnik, D. B. (1997). Stigma. *Webster's new world college dictionary* (3rd ed.). New York: Macmillan.

Newman, M. (2006, July 26). Yates found not guilty by reason of insanity. *The New York Times.* Retrieved from http://www.nytimes.com/2006/07/26/us/26cnd-yates.html?_r=1&

Nonacs, R. (2007). *A deeper shade of blue: A woman's guide to recognizing and treating depression in her childbearing years* (1st trade paperback ed.). New York: Simon & Schuster.

Office on Women's Health, U.S. Department of Health and Human Services. (2012, July 16). *Hashimoto's disease fact sheet.* Retrieved from http://www.womenshealth.gov/publications/our-publications/fact-sheet/hashimoto-disease.html#a

Paul, M. (2013, March 13). *Surprising rate of women have depression after childbirth.* Northwestern University. Retrieved from http://www.northwestern.edu/newscenter/stories/2013/03/surprising-rate-of-women-have-depression-after-childbirth.html

Paulson, J. F., & Bazemore, S. D. (2010). Prenatal and postpartum depression in fathers and its association with maternal depression: A meta-analysis. *Journal of the American Medical Association, 303*(19), 1961-1969. doi:10.1001/jama.2010.605

Postpartum Men. (n.d.). *Men's depression.* Retrieved from http://www.postpartummen.com/depression.htm

Postpartum Men. (n.d.). *Postpartum depression.* Retrieved from http://www.postpartummen.com/postpartum-depression.htm

Postpartum Support International. (n.d.). *Anxiety during pregnancy and postpartum.* Retrieved from http://www.postpartum.net/learn-more/anxiety-during-pregnancy-postpartum/

Postpartum Support International. (n.d.). *Depression during pregnancy and postpartum.* Retrieved from http://www.postpartum.net/learn-more/depression-during-pregnancy-postpartum/

Postpartum Support International. (n.d.). *Postpartum post-traumatic stress disorder.* Retrieved from http://www.postpartum.net/learn-more/postpartum-post-traumatic-stress-disorder/

Postpartum Support International. (n.d.). *Postpartum psychosis.* Retrieved from http://www.postpartum.net/learn-more/postpartum-psychosis/

Postpartum Support International. (n.d.). *Pregnancy and postpartum mental health.* Retrieved from http://www.postpartum.net/learn-more/pregnancy-postpartum-mental-health/

Postpartum Support International. (n.d.). *Pregnancy or postpartum obsessive symptoms.* Retrieved from http://www.postpartum.net/learn-more/pregnancy-or-postpartum-obsessive-symptoms/

Rhodes, G. (2015, November 23). Is perinatal anxiety a bigger problem than postnatal depression? *The Guardian.* Retrieved from http://www.theguardian.com/lifeandstyle/2015/nov/23/perinatal-anxiety-postnatal-depression

Segre, L. S., & Davis, W. N. (2013, June). *Postpartum depression and perinatal mood disorders in the DSM*. Retrieved from http://www.postpartum.net/wp-content/uploads/2014/11/DSM-5-Summary-PSI.pdf

Shomon, M. (2017). *Hypothyroidism and pregnancy: Frequently asked questions about being pregnant with an underactive thyroid*. Retrieved from http://www.thyroid-info.com/articles/pregnancy.htm

Silberner, J. (2016, January 26). Depression screening recommended for all pregnant women, new mothers. *NPR*. Retrieved from http://www.npr.org/sections/health-shots/2016/01/26/464415212/depression-screening-recommended-for-all-pregnant-women-new-mothers

Sittser, J. (2004). *A grace disguised: How the soul grows through loss*. Grand Rapids, MI: Zondervan.

Stone, K. (n.d.). *Meet Katherine Stone*. Retrieved from http://fierceandpowerful.com/wordpress/meet-katherine-stone

Stone, K. (2013, March 15). *Postpartum depression is [not] surprisingly more common* [Blog post]. Retrieved from http://www.postpartumprogress.com/postpartum-depression-is-not-surprisingly-more-common

Tartakovsky, M. (2016). *5 damaging myths about postpartum depression*. Retrieved from http://psychcentral.com/lib/5-damaging-myths-about-postpartum-depression/

Tchividjian, T. (2012). *Glorious ruin: How suffering sets you free*. Colorado Springs, CO: David C Cook.

Tel Aviv University. (2014, July 8). *TAU study on interrupted sleep*. Retrieved from https://english.tau.ac.il/news/tau_study_interrupted_sleep

The Postpartum Stress Center. (2010). *Are you having thoughts that are scaring you?* Retrieved from http://postpartumstress.com/admin/wp-content/uploads/2012/02/ScaryThoughts-1.pdf

Thurgood, S., Avery, D. M., & Williamson, L. (2009). Postpartum depression (PPD). *American Journal of Clinical Medicine, 6*(2), 17-22. Retrieved from http://www.aapsus.org/articles/11.pdf

Twomey, T. M. (2009). *Understanding postpartum psychosis: A temporary madness*. Westport, CT: Praeger.

University of North Carolina. (n.d.). *What is the 4th trimester project?* Retrieved from http://4thtrimester.web.unc.edu/2015/12/31/4th-trimester/

University of North Carolina Press. (n.d.). *Author Q&A: Judith Walzer Leavitt, author of Make room for daddy: The journey from waiting room to birthing* room, delivers an account of the evolving role of fathers in childbirth. Retrieved from http://www.uncpress.unc.edu/browse/page/572

U.S. Congresswoman Katherine Clark. (2016). *Clark praises plan to ensure coverage for postpartum depression* [Press release]. Retrieved from http://katherineclark.house.gov/index.cfm/ press-releases?ID=7A626B0C-BA68-48B5-81E0-D7B5C19F76D5

U.S. Preventive Services Task Force. (2016). *U.S. Preventive Services Task Force recommends clinicians screen all adults for depression* [Press release]. Retrieved from https://www.uspreventiveservicestaskforce.org/ Home/GetFile/6/250/depressionadultsfinalbulletin/pdf

Weiss, R. E. (2016, April 28). *How is pitocin used to induce labor?* Retrieved from https://www.verywell.com/how-is-pitocin-used-to-induce-labor-2758964

Whitlock, S. (2015, December 4). *CNN insanity: Erin Burnett wonders if 'postpartum psychosis' led to slaughter* [Blog post]. Retrieved from http://www.newsbusters.org/blogs/nb/scott-whitlock/2015/12/04/ cnn-stunner-erin-burnett-asks-if-postpartum-psychosis-led#sthash. cq5Uon7P.dpuf

Wisner, K. L., Sit, D. K. Y., McShea, M. C., Rizzo, D. M., Zoretich, R. A., Hughes, C. L. ... Hanusa, B. H. (2013). Onset timing, thoughts of self-harm, and diagnoses in postpartum women with screen-positive depression findings. *Journal of the American Medical Association/Psychiatry, 70*(5), 490-498. doi:10.1001/jamapsychiatry.2013.87

Yancey, P. (2009). *Grace.* Retrieved from http://philipyancey. com/q-and-a-topics/

Index